D1757422

Intravenous Infusions
a guide to their calculation

Simon B Poole, MBBS

RADCLIFFE MEDICAL PRESS
OXFORD

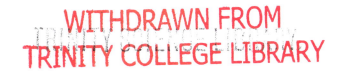

© 1990 Radcliffe Medical Press Ltd
15 Kings Meadow, Ferry Hinksey Road, Oxford OX2 0DP

British Library Cataloguing in Publication Data
Poole, Simon, 1963-
Intravenous infusions, a guide to their calculation.
1. Man. Intravenous therapy. Infusion
I. Title
615.6
ISBN 1 870905 71 7

Printed in Great Britain by Billing & Sons Ltd, Worcester
Typeset by Advance Typesetting Ltd, Oxfordshire

CONTENTS

FOREWORD

The author is to be congratulated for compiling in a straightforward, simple and easily comprehensible style the vital information that is necessary to infuse drugs by the intravenous route. Even the simplest calculations when undertaken under the circumstance of sleeplessness or duress may be performed incorrectly and dosage errors in such circumstances may lead to serious adverse consequences. To have available a readily accessible guide to the calculation of dosage for intravenous infusions will be a great help to junior doctors and to nursing staff. If reference to this book improves the accuracy of dosing and reduces the incidence of adverse drug reactions then it will have achieved an important goal.

PETER S SEVER
Professor of Clinical Pharmacology
St Marys Hospital Medical School

INTRODUCTION

This guide to the calculation of intravenous infusions has been compiled primarily to help and reassure junior doctors, nurses and pharmacists involved in their prescription.

In my experience as a junior doctor many drugs requiring infusion are used in situations of acute illness, where rapid administration may have great prognostic implications. The *British National Formulary* (BNF) and drug data sheets, whilst providing much invaluable information, rarely demonstrate examples of the mathematics used to translate units such as micrograms per kilogram body-weight per minute into a practical number of millilitres of dilute infusion solution per hour.

Calculations usually involve fairly straightforward theory, but difficulties arise on occasions demanding quick decisions from a doctor who may be significantly sleep deprived. A simple mathematical mistake in prescription can easily lead to tenfold or one hundredfold errors in dose administration with possible disastrous medical consequence. This is every junior doctor's nightmare, and out of this was born the idea for this guide.

Information contained here is not exhaustive and the aim of this handbook is to provide a source of reference. It is recommended that it be used in conjunction with the BNF and data sheets, and as a confirmation and reassurance that the prescriber's own calculations approximate to those given here. Where dose is specifically weight-related, 60 kg is taken as an average reference figure. Certain regimens, such as cytotoxic drugs and anaesthetic drugs, in addition to paediatric doses are beyond the scope of this guide, and the reader should in these instances seek specialist advice.

Dilutions usually involve 500 ml bags of fluid, and small amounts of drug diluent may be omitted from calculations when judged insignificant. In certain circumstances the author accepts that smaller or larger fluid loads may be required according to clinical demand (e.g. in cases of cardiac failure) and regimens should be adjusted accordingly. 0.9% saline and 5% dextrose are used in the example infusions, but other fluids may also be compatible. No information regarding life of infusions is included.

Accompanying each dose calculation is a reminder of indications, contraindications, precautions, side-effects and drug interactions to provide a quick source of reference. No distinction has been made between contraindications and precautions since in clinical practice it is often impossible to adhere to strict guidelines when benefits might outweigh risks.

I should like to take this opportunity to thank the manufacturers of the products included in the guide for their advice and corrections, Dr. Richard Needle for his painstaking proofreading, Radcliffe Medical Press and, finally, my wife for continual encouragement.

SIMON B POOLE
August, 1990

ACETYLCYSTEINE

Proprietary Name

▽ Parvolex (Duncan, Flockhart and Co. Ltd)

Indications

▽ Paracetamol overdose (seek expert advice from nearest Poisons
Unit (*see* Appendix 1)). Blood paracetamol levels must be taken
at least 4 hours after overdose to determine if treatment threshold
has been passed. Liver function may be best monitored by
regular clotting tests. Most active within 8 hours of ingestion.
Not for administration more than 15 hours after overdose.

Contraindications and Precautions

▽ Care in asthma
▽ Pregnancy

Side-effects

▽ Anaphylaxis
▽ Rashes   } Usually in first 15–60 minutes of infusion

Presentation

▽ Clear, colourless solution
▽ Ampoule of 2 g in 10 ml (200 mg/ml)

Dosage as Parvolex

In first 15 minutes infuse at 150 mg/kg
Mix (e.g.) 150 mg × 60 kg = 9 g (4½ ampoules = 45 ml)
Infuse in 200 ml 5% dextrose over 15 minutes

Then infuse at a rate of 50 mg/kg for 4 hours
Mix (e.g.) 50 mg × 60 kg = 3 g (1½ ampoules) in 500 ml
5% dextrose
Infuse in 4 hours at 125 ml per hour

For further 16 hours infuse at 100 mg/kg
Mix (e.g.) 100 mg × 60 kg = 6 g (3 ampoules) in 1 litre
5% dextrose
Infuse over 16 hours at 64 ml per hour

ACYCLOVIR

Proprietary Name

▽ Zovirax (Wellcome Medical Division)

Indications

▽ *Herpes simplex* and *Varicella zoster*, especially in the immunocompromised
▽ Herpes encephalitis

Contraindications and Precautions

▽ Hypersensitivity
▽ Impaired renal function
▽ Pregnancy (but may be used in chickenpox dissemination of pregnancy)

Side-effects

▽ Increase in blood urea and creatinine levels
▽ Rarely renal failure
▽ Rashes
▽ Increases in liver-related enzymes have been reported
▽ Decreases in haematological indices have been reported
▽ Neurological reactions including tremor and confusion
▽ Gastrointestinal disturbances

Drug Interactions

▽ Probenecid increases acyclovir half-life

Presentation

▽ White to off-white powder
▽ Vials of 250 mg and 500 mg for reconstitution

Dosage as Zovirax

In immunocompetent with recurrent *Varicella* or *Herpes simplex* infection, and immunocompromised with *Herpes simplex* 5 mg/kg tds

In immunocompromised and/or cases of encephalitis, increase dose to 10 mg/kg tds

Dose must be altered if renal function is impaired (*see* specialist literature)

Maximum concentration of 5 mg acyclovir per ml solution (e.g.) for 5 mg/kg dose in 60 kg adult
Reconstitute 2 × 250 mg or 1 × 500 mg vial with 20 ml 0.9% saline or water for injections
Mix 12 ml (= 300 mg) to 100–250 ml 0.9% saline and infuse over 1 hour

For 10 mg/kg dose in 60 kg adult
Reconstitute 3 × 250 mg vials with 30 ml 0.9% saline or water for injections
Mix 24 ml (= 600 mg) with 250 ml 0.9% saline and infuse over 1 hour

ALTEPLASE (rt-PA)

Proprietary Name

▽ Actilyse (Boehringer Ingelheim)

Indications

▽ Fibrinolytic therapy of acute thrombotic coronary artery
occlusion. Treatment should be initiated within 6 hours of
onset of chest pain

Contraindications and Precautions

▽ History of cerebrovascular disease or uncontrolled hypertension
▽ Bleeding diathesis and severe liver disease
▽ Within 10 days of severe internal bleeding, major surgery or trauma
▽ Any potential bleeding site including active peptic ulceration,
acute pancreatitis, ulcerative colitis, visceral carcinoma,
diabetic retinopathy, etc.
▽ Bacterial endocarditis
▽ Pregnancy

Side-effects

▽ Haemorrhage including CVA
▽ Reperfusion arrhythmias
▽ Nausea and vomiting

Drug Interactions

▽ Any drug affecting coagulation will affect pharmacodynamics
▽ Consider use of heparin following administration and the use of
long-term oral aspirin following myocardial infarction

Presentation

▽ Powder
▽ Vial of 50 mg (29,000,000 IU) with diluent (50 ml), transfer device and infusion bag = 1 mg/ml

Dosage as Actilyse

Recommended dose of 100 mg (2 vials ≡ 58 million IU) in 3 hours

First inject 10 mg (10 ml = ⅕ vial) as bolus over 1–2 minutes
Then mix 50 mg (50 ml = 1 vial) in 100–250 ml 0.9% saline (the only recommended diluent) and infuse over 1 hour

Then mix 40 mg (40 ml = ⅘ vial) with 100–250 ml 0.9% saline and infuse over 2 hours

AMIODARONE HYDROCHLORIDE

Proprietary Name

▽ Cordarone X (Sanofi UK Ltd)

Indications

▽ Wolff-Parkinson-White syndrome associated tachyarrhythmias
▽ Supraventricular nodal and ventricular tachycardias*
▽ Atrial fibrillation and flutter*
▽ Recurrent ventricular fibrillation*

* Where other drugs are ineffective or contraindicated. Injection to be used where a rapid response is required. Tablets are used for stabilization and long-term treatment

Contraindications and Precautions

▽ Circulatory collapse or severe arterial hypotension
▽ Sinus bradycardia
▽ Atrioventricular block
▽ Thyroid dysfunction
▽ Pregnancy and lactation
▽ Iodine sensitivity
▽ Latent or manifest heart failure
▽ Porphyria

Side-effects

Mainly associated with long-term oral administration

▽ Corneal deposits
▽ Photosensitivity rash
▽ Thyroid dysfunction
▽ Diffuse pulmonary alveolitis
▽ Peripheral neuropathy
▽ Hepatotoxicity
▽ Nausea and vomiting
▽ Ataxia

Drug Interactions

▽ Digoxin
▽ Oral anticoagulants
▽ Phenytoin or other highly protein-bound drugs
▽ Calcium antagonists and beta-blockers may potentiate bradycardia

Presentation

▽ Clear, pale-yellow solution
▽ Ampoule of 150 mg in 3 ml

Dosage as Cordarone X via caval catheter

5 mg/kg over 20 minutes–2 hours
(e.g.) 60 kg adult
5 mg × 60 kg = 300 mg
Mix 2 × 150 mg ampoules with 250 ml 5% dextrose
(the only recommended solution)
Infuse over 20 minutes–2 hours

This may be followed by repeat infusions up to 1200 mg
(approximately 15 mg/kg) in up to 500 ml 5% dextrose in
24 hours. In extreme clinical emergency, the drug may, at the
clinician's discretion, be given as a slow injection of 150–300 mg
in 10–20 ml 5% dextrose over 1–2 minutes, the patient being
closely monitored, e.g. in an intensive care unit.

AMPHOTERICIN

Proprietary Name

▽ Fungizone (Bristol-Myers Squibb Pharmaceuticals Ltd)

Indications

▽ Systemic fungal infections

Contraindications and Precautions

▽ Hypersensitivity
▽ Liver or renal dysfunction
▽ Blood dyscrasias
▽ Pregnancy

Side-effects

▽ Fever and malaise
▽ Headache
▽ Gastrointestinal symptoms
▽ Muscle and joint pains
▽ Thrombophlebitis
▽ Hypokalaemia
▽ Anaemia
▽ Renal damage
▽ Rarely arrhythmias, blood dyscrasias, acute liver failure,
   neurological symptoms (including vertigo, tinnitus, diplopia,
   convulsions and neuropathy)

Drug Interactions

▽ Increased risk of nephrotoxicity with aminoglycosides,
   cyclosporin and cephalothin
▽ Antagonism by miconazole
▽ Diuretics and corticosteroids may potentiate hypokalaemia

Presentation

▽ Yellow, fluffy powder
▽ Vial of 50 mg for reconstitution with 10 ml = 5 mg/ml

Dosage as Fungizone

Mix required amount of the concentrate with 500 ml 5% dextrose as follows:

For starting dose of 250 µg/kg per day
250 × 60 = 15000 µg = 15 mg
Therefore, mix 3 ml solution with 500 ml 5% dextrose

Infuse over 6 hours

Increase dose gradually to 1 mg/kg per day
1 × 60 = 60 mg per day
Therefore, mix 10 ml (1 vial) + 2 ml from second vial with 500 ml 5% dextrose
Maximum recommended dose of 1.5 mg/kg per day

ATENOLOL

Proprietary Name

▽ Tenormin (Stuart Pharmaceuticals Ltd)

Indications

▽ Management of cardiac dysrhythmias (rarely first-line treatment)
▽ Some evidence to show that early intervention in myocardial infarction reduces infarct size, decreases incidence of ventricular arrhythmias and provides analgesia. However, intravenous atenolol is not used routinely in myocardial infarction

Contraindications and Precautions

▽ Second or third degree heart block
▽ Cardiogenic shock
▽ Care in cardiac failure
▽ Obstructive airways disease and asthma
▽ Renal failure
▽ Peripheral vascular disease
▽ Pregnancy
▽ Diabetes: atenolol modifies some signs of hypoglycaemia

Side-effects

▽ Myocardial depression including cardiac failure
▽ Bradycardia
▽ Bronchospasm
▽ Peripheral vasoconstriction
▽ Muscular fatigue

Drug Interactions

▽ Other antiarrhythmics especially Class I types
(e.g. disopyramide) may potentiate myocardial depression,
bradycardias and AV block
▽ Hypotensives – calcium antagonists, including verapamil, may
induce severe hypotension and cardiac failure, and should not
be combined with atenolol especially in patients with impaired
ventricular function. Verapamil and beta-blockers should not be
administered within 24 hours of each other
▽ Antidiabetic drugs may have an increased hypoglycaemic effect,
signs of which may be masked by beta-blockade

Presentation

▽ Clear, colourless solution
▽ Ampoule of 5 mg in 10 ml = 0.5 mg/ml

Dosage as Tenormin

Injected intravenously as single dose of 2.5 mg (5 ml) over 2½ minutes (i.e. 1 mg per minute)
May be repeated at 5 minute intervals until response is observed up to a maximum of 10 mg

Infusion at dose of 150 µg/kg body-weight
(e.g.) 60 kg adult needs 9 mg = 18 ml = 1⅘ ampoules

Mix in 100 ml of 5% dextrose or 0.9% saline and infuse over 20 minutes
May be repeated, if required, every 12 hours

CEPHRADINE AND CEFTIZOXIME

Proprietary Names

▽ Velosef (Bristol-Myers Squibb Pharmaceuticals Ltd)
▽ Cefizox (Wellcome Medical Division)

Indications

▽ Infection due to sensitive Gram-positive and Gram-negative bacteria
▽ Includes urinary and respiratory tract infections, skin, bone and soft-tissue infections
▽ Surgical prophylaxis

Contraindications and Precautions

▽ Hypersensitivity to cephalosporins
▽ Hypersensitivity to penicillins
▽ Pregnancy and lactation
▽ Renal impairment
▽ False positive urinary stick tests and Coomb's test
▽ Porphyria

Side-effects

▽ Allergic reactions
▽ Gastrointestinal symptoms

Drug Interactions

▽ Probenicid reduces excretion

Presentation

▽ Velosef: Powder
  Cefizox: White to pale-yellow powder
▽ Velosef: Vials of 500 mg and 1 g to be reconstituted with
  5 and 10 ml respectively = 100 mg/ml
  Cefizox: Vials of 500 mg, 1 g and 2 g to be reconstituted with
  2, 3 and 6 ml respectively = 250 mg/ml, 333 mg/ml

Dosage as Velosef (cephradine)

Dose of 500 mg qds or 1 g bd up to 8 g daily

Mix 500 mg with 100 ml 0.9% saline or 5% dextrose
Infuse over 50–100 minutes

Dosage as Cefizox (cefizoxime)

Up to 8 g daily

0.5–1 g bd (increased in severe infections)
Similar solution: mix as above

CHLORAMPHENICOL

Proprietary Name

▽ Kemicetine (Farmitalia Carlo Erba Ltd)

Indications

▽ Severe infections due to susceptible organisms. These include many Gram-negative and Gram-positive bacteria, spirillae and rickettsia
▽ Especially useful in epiglottitis and children with meningitis likely to be due to *Haemophilus influenzae* infections

Contraindications and Precautions

▽ Porphyria
▽ Pregnancy and breast-feeding
▽ Hepatic impairment

Side-effects

▽ Blood dyscrasias
▽ Optic or peripheral neuritis
▽ Gastrointestinal symptoms
▽ Fungal superinfections
▽ Erythema multiforme
▽ 'Grey syndrome'

Drug Interactions

▽ Potentiation of oral anticoagulants, sulphonylureas and phenytoin
▽ Rifampicin and barbiturates increase metabolism of chloramphenicol

Presentation

▽ Powder
▽ Vial of 1 g for reconstitution

Dosage as Kemicetine

(May be given by slow intravenous injection)

Daily dose of 50 mg/kg
Therefore, for 60 kg adult = 50 × 60 = 3000 mg per day in divided doses
Therefore, give infusion of 1 g chloramphenicol every 8 hours

Mix one ampoule in 100–250 ml 0.9% saline or 5% dextrose
Infuse over 30–60 minutes

CHLORMETHIAZOLE

Proprietary Name

▽ Heminevrin 0.8% infusion (Astra Pharmaceuticals Ltd)

Indications

▽ Acute alcohol withdrawal
▽ To sedate
▽ Anticonvulsant in status epilepticus and pre-eclamptic toxaemia

Contraindications and Precautions

▽ Hypersensitivity
▽ Acute pulmonary insufficiency
▽ Pregnancy especially in the first trimester
▽ Lactation
▽ Hepatic and renal dysfunction
▽ Cardiac and respiratory disease
  N.B. Close observation is imperative, since induced sedation can pass unnoticed into deep unconsciousness, with subsequent risk of mechanical airway obstruction

Side-effects

▽ Sneezing
▽ Conjunctival irritation
▽ Headache
▽ Hypotension
▽ Respiratory depression
▽ Gastrointestinal disturbances
▽ Local thrombophlebitis
▽ Confusion

Drug Interactions

▽ Cimetidine inhibits metabolism
▽ Potentiated by other CNS depressants

Presentation

▽ Colourless, aqueous solution
▽ 500 ml bottle of chlormethiazole edisylate 8 mg/ml (0.8%)
   containing 4 g in total

Dosage as Heminevrin

Dose in status epilepticus

40–100 ml over 5–10 minutes will usually stop convulsion.
Thereafter a reduced dose should be titrated against clinical
response

Dose in acute alcohol withdrawal

Similar to above

Dose in pre-eclampsia where it is necessary to sedate and
raise the threshold for convulsions

Start at a rate of 4 ml per minute for approximately 10 minutes
(until the onset of drowsiness)
Thereafter maintenance dose typically of 0.5–1 ml per min
(30–60 ml per hour)

CIMETIDINE AND RANITIDINE

Proprietary Name

▽ Tagamet (SmithKline Beecham)
▽ Zantac (Glaxo)

Indications

▽ Duodenal and benign gastric ulceration
▽ Stomal ulceration (only cimetidine)
▽ Oesophageal reflux syndrome
▽ Zollinger-Ellison syndrome
▽ Prophylaxis of gastrointestinal haemorrhage from stress ulceration in seriously ill patients
▽ Prevention of acid aspiration syndrome
▽ Other conditions where reduction in gastric acid is beneficial e.g. malabsorption, pancreatic insufficiency

Contraindications and Precautions

▽ Hypersensitivity
▽ Renal and hepatic impairment
▽ Pregnancy and lactation

Side-effects

▽ Diarrhoea
▽ Dizziness
▽ Rash
▽ Gynaecomastia with swelling and tenderness
▽ Reversible liver damage
▽ Reversible confusional states
▽ Nephritis, blood dyscrasias, acute pancreatitis, muscle and joint pains have been reported very rarely. Cardiac arrhythmias have been reported very rarely, possibly associated with rapid intravenous injection

Drug Interactions

▽ Cimetidine increases plasma levels of the following drugs:

Opioid analgesics
Lignocaine*
Procainamide and flecainide
Metronidazole
Oral anticoagulants*
Antidepressants
Calcium-channel blockers
Beta-blockers
Benzodiazepines
Chloroquine
Metformin
Phenytoin and carbamazepine*
Theophylline*

▽ Ranitidine probably has less potential to react with other drugs

The clinical significance of these interactions varies greatly but the more important ones have been asterisked

Presentation as Tagamet (cimetidine)

▽ Clear, colourless liquid
▽ Supplied as 400 mg cimetidine in 100 ml 0.9% solution or
200 mg in 2 ml ampoule = 100 mg/ml for mixing as above

Dosage as Tagamet (cimetidine)

Recommended dose of 200–400 mg every 4 to 6 hours or
20–30 mg/kg per day in divided dose
Infuse 100 ml over 30–60 minutes

Continuous infusion should be at a rate of 50–100 mg per hour
over 24 hours (e.g. 66 mg per hour = 1600 mg in 24 hours)
Therefore infuse 100 ml (400 mg) cimetidine solution over
6 hours at a rate of 16 ml per hour

Presentation as Zantac (ranitidine)

▽ Clear, colourless liquid
▽ Ampoule of 50 mg in 2 ml = 25 mg/ml

Dosage as Zantac (ranitidine)

Mix 1 ampoule with 100 ml or 250 ml 0.9% saline or 5% dextrose
Infuse over 2 hours at a rate of 25 mg per hour
Repeat infusion every 6 to 8 hours

In prophylaxis of upper gastrointestinal haemorrhage from stress
ulcer in the severely ill patient the manufacturer recommends
continuous infusion of 0.125–0.25 mg/kg per hour following a
50 mg priming dose as a slow injection
(e.g.) 0.25 × 60 kg = 15 mg per hour
Mix 50 mg in 500 ml 0.9% saline or 5% dextrose
1 mg in 10 ml
Therefore, infuse at 150 ml per hour

COLISTIN

Proprietary Name

▽ Colomycin (Pharmax Ltd) (colistin sulphomethate sodium)

Indications

▽ Infections by susceptible Gram-negative organisms including *Pseudomonas aeruginosa* and *Klebsiella*

   Toxicity usually limits systemic use to severe infections or septicaemias, often where other antibiotics have been unsuccessful

Contraindications and Precautions

▽ Hypersensitivity to colistin
▽ Myasthenia gravis
▽ Pregnancy and lactation

Side-effects

▽ Nephrotoxicity (usually reversible)
▽ Facial paraesthesiae and vertigo
▽ Slurred speech, visual disturbances, confusion or psychosis
▽ Muscle weakness and apnoea

   The above effects only usually occur in overdosage or where no adjustment to dose has been made to allow for impaired renal function

Drug Interactions

▽ Colistin increases effects of curariform muscle relaxants
▽ Side-effects and nephrotoxicity may be increased with concomitant use of other nephrotoxic drugs e.g. aminoglycosides

Presentation

▽ Creamy-white powder
▽ Vials of 500,000 units and 1,000,000 units for reconstitution

Dosage as Colomycin

Ampoules of 500,000 units or 1,000,000 units

Dose for 60 kg adult with normal renal function (may be increased if clinically indicated)
6,000,000 units per 24 hours
i.e. 3,000,000 units twice a day

Mix 3 × 1,000,000 ampoules in 500 ml 0.9% saline or 5% dextrose

Infuse for a minimum of 1 hour, maximum of 6 hours

CO-TRIMOXAZOLE

Proprietary Name

▽ Bactrim (Roche Products Ltd)
▽ Septrin (Wellcome)

Indications

▽ Invasive *Salmonella*
▽ Exacerbation of chronic bronchitis
▽ Bone and joint infections due to *Haemophilus influenzae*
▽ Gonorrhoea in penicillin-sensitive patients
▽ Urinary tract infections
▽ Typhoid fever
▽ *Pneumocystis carinii*: where the oral route of administration is inappropriate

Contraindications and Precautions

▽ Hypersensitivity to sulphonomides or trimethroprim
▽ Infants under 6 weeks of age
▽ Liver dysfunction
▽ Renal insufficiency
▽ Glucose-6-phosphate dehydrogenase deficiency
▽ Blood dyscrasias
▽ Elderly
▽ Pregnancy
▽ Folate deficiency

Side-effects

▽ Hypersensitivity
▽ Gastrointestinal symptoms
▽ Erythema multiforme
▽ Blood dyscrasias
▽ Megaloblastic anaemias
▽ Allergic skin reactions
▽ Pulmonary infiltrates

Drug Interactions

▽ Enhances effect of thiopentone, oral anticoagulants, oral
  hypoglycaemics, phenytoin
▽ Increased risk of reversible kidney damage with cyclosporin
▽ Increased risk of folate deficiency with methotrexate (also
  increases free methotrexate levels in blood) and anti-malarial
  drugs
▽ Increased risk of thrombocytopenia with certain diuretics
  (e.g. thiazides)

Presentation as Bactrim or Septrin

▽ Colourless to slightly-yellow liquid
▽ Ampoule of 480 mg in 5 ml (96 mg/ml)

Dosage as Bactrim or Septrin

Usual dose of 960 mg bd given as ampoules diluted in 250 ml solution twice a day

Maximum dose (for severe infections) = 1440 mg bd
Dilute 3 ampoules in 500 ml 5% dextrose or 0.9% saline
Infuse over 90 minutes

The maximum dose can be given for maximum of three successive days by intravenous route

Higher than 'maximum' dose may be required for treatment of *Pneumocystis*. Facilities for regular monitoring of drug levels and renal function are recommended. Dose may require reduction if renal function poor. NB In high dose solutions may need to be more concentrated

120 mg/kg per day (e.g.) 60 kg adult = 7200 mg per day
= 1800 mg qds

See table below

Patient weight in kg	6-hourly dose co-trimoxazole in mg	ml solution *(before dilution in infusion)*	No. of ampoules
48	1440	15	3
51.2	1536	16	
54.4	1632	17	
57.6	1728	18	
60.8	1824	19	
64	1920	20	4
67.2	2016	21	
70.4	2112	22	
73.6	2208	23	
76.8	2304	24	
80 kg	2400	25	5

DESFERRIOXAMINE MESYLATE

Proprietary Name

▽ Desferal (Ciba Laboratories)

Indications

▽ Acute iron poisoning
▽ Primary and secondary haemochromatosis including thalassaemia

Contraindications and Precautions

▽ Hypersensitivity
▽ Care in renal disease
▽ Use with prochlorperazine may result in prolonged unconsciousness
▽ Pregnancy

Side-effects

▽ Anaphylaxis
▽ Hypotension especially when administered too rapidly
▽ Dizziness or convulsions
▽ Gastrointestinal disturbances
▽ Renal and hepatic impairment (possibly effect of iron or iron desferrioxamine complex)
▽ Visual and hearing disturbances
▽ Red/brown discoloration of urine

Drug Interactions

▽ Prochlorperazine – *see* above

Presentation

▽ Powder
▽ Vial of 500 mg for reconstitution with 5 ml = 100 mg/ml

Dosage as Desferal

Not for direct intravenous injection
In acute iron poisoning

Theoretically, 100 mg desferrioxamine chelates approximately
8.5 mg of iron. Therefore, 5 g desferrioxamine chelates
approximately 10 ferrous sulphate tablets

For infusion in emergency seek expert advice (*see* Appendix 1 for
nearest Poisons Unit)

In thalassaemia
See data sheet for full details
20–40 mg/kg over 8–12 hours
Dosage should be adjusted to suit individual patient
(e.g.) 60 kg adult 1.2–2.4 g in 1 litre 5% dextrose or 0.9% saline
over 8–12 hours

DIAZEPAM

Proprietary Name

▽ Diazemuls (Dumex Pharmaceuticals)
▽ Diazepam Injection (Stesolid) (CP Pharmaceuticals Ltd)
▽ Valium (Roche Products Ltd)

Indications

▽ Severe acute anxiety or agitation
▽ Control of convulsions, status epilepticus
▽ Tetanus
▽ Delirium tremens
▽ Acute muscle spasm
▽ Pre-operative medication or premedication

Contraindications and Precautions

▽ Hypersensitivity to benzodiazepines
▽ Pulmonary insufficiency and respiratory depression
▽ Myasthenia gravis
▽ Porphyria
▽ Elderly (reduce dose)
▽ Phobic or obsessional states
▽ Chronic psychosis
▽ Organic brain disease

Side-effects

▽ Unsteadiness and ataxia
▽ Drowsiness and sedation
▽ Respiratory depression
▽ Confusion
▽ Rare adverse effects include headache, vertigo, hypotension, gastrointestinal upsets, skin rashes, visual disturbances, changes in libido, urinary retention

Drug Interactions

▽ Potentiates effects of other CNS depressants
▽ Cimetidine decreases clearance
▽ Phenobarbitone increases clearance
▽ Disulfiram

Presentation of Diazemuls

▽ White, opaque emulsion
▽ Ampoules of 10 mg in 2 ml = 5 mg/ml

Presentation of Diazepam Injection (Stesolid)

▽ Clear, colourless to yellow solution
▽ Ampoules of 10 mg in 2 ml = 5 mg/ml

Presentation of Valium

▽ Greenish-yellow solution
▽ Ampoules of 10 mg in 2 ml = 5 mg/ml

Dosage as Diazemuls, Diazepam Injection (Stesolid) or Valium

Diazemuls should be diluted with 5% or 10% dextrose
Stesolid or Valium should be diluted with 5% dextrose or
0.9% saline
Dosage and administration depends on indication

Infusion may follow bolus injection of 10–20 mg over
2 minutes
Repeated after 30–60 minutes if necessary

Infuse to a maximum rate of 3 mg/kg over 24 hours for status
epilepticus, convulsions due to poisoning and tetanus
(the dose in the latter may occasionally exceed this)
Therefore, maximum of 180 mg over 24 hours
(e.g.) 40 mg in 500 ml over 6 hours × 4 = 160 mg in 2 litres
total per day
N.B. This is near maximum dose

The manufacturers of Stesolid and Valium recommend maximum
concentrations of 25 and 40 mg respectively in 500 ml diluent
Doses should be adjusted accordingly

DIGOXIN

Proprietary Name

▽ Lanoxin (Wellcome Medical Division)

Indications

▽ Supraventricular arrhythmias, particularly atrial fibrillation
  IV infusion recommended where rapid digitalization required

Contraindications and Precautions

▽ Supraventricular arrhythmias caused by Wolff-Parkinson-White
  syndrome
▽ Care in elderly
▽ Recent myocardial infarction
▽ Renal impairment
▽ Avoid hypokalaemia
▽ Hypercalcaemia
▽ Hypothyroidism
▽ Previous recent or concurrent digoxin therapy

Side-effects

▽ Gastrointestinal symptoms
▽ Visual disturbances
▽ CNS disturbances
▽ Cardiac arrhythmias

Drug Interactions

▽ NSAIDs may exacerbate heart failure and reduce clearance
▽ Amiodarone and quinidine increase digoxin concentrations
▽ Erythromycin enhances effect of digoxin
▽ Quinidine increases digoxin concentrations
▽ Suxamethonium, beta-blockers, verapamil may increase
  arrhythmias, bradycardia or AV block
▽ Digoxin toxicity may worsen with potassium-losing diuretics

Presentation as Lanoxin

▽ Clear, colourless solution
▽ Ampoules of 500 µg in 2 ml = 250 µg/ml

Dosage as Lanoxin

Dose of 0.75 to 1 mg in 50–100 ml 5% dextrose or 0.9% saline over ½–1 hour

Then normal maintenance therapy
If patient has been on oral digoxin previously, IV dose should be about 30% less

DISODIUM ETIDRONATE

Proprietary Name

▽ Didronel IV (Norwich Eaton Ltd)

Indications

▽ Hypercalcaemia of malignancy with or without bone metastasis, when other modes of therapy, such as hydration have inadequately reduced elevated serum calcium

(It is most important that hydration be attended to in the first line treatment of hypercalcaemia)

Contraindications and Precautions

▽ Hypersensitivity to disodium etidronate
▽ Impaired renal function where serum creatinine is greater than 440 µmol/l
▽ Pregnancy

Side-effects

▽ Alteration in taste sensation
▽ Possible further impairment of compromised renal function
▽ Possible symptoms of hypocalcaemia in overdose

Presentation as Didronel IV

▽ Clear, colourless solution
▽ Ampoule of 300 mg in 6 ml = 50 mg/ml

Dosage as Didronel IV

Recommended 3 day course of 7.5 mg/kg per day

7.5 mg × 60 kg = 450 mg
Therefore, 1 ampoule = 6 ml = 300 mg
+ ½ ampoule = 3 ml = 150 mg

Mix 1½ ampoules (9 ml) in minimum of 250 ml 0.9% saline
Infuse over minimum period of 2 hours

Monitor electrolyte and calcium responses closely

DISODIUM PAMIDRONATE

Proprietary Name

▽ Aredia (Ciba Laboratories)

Indications

▽ Hypercalcaemia induced by tumours
   (It is most important that hydration be attended to in the first
   line treatment of hypercalcaemia)

Contraindications and Precautions

▽ Hypersensitivity to disodium pamidronate
▽ Severe renal impairment
▽ Possibility of precipitating convulsions in some patients due
   to changes in electrolytes
▽ Children and pregnancy

Side-effects

▽ Mild transient rise in body temperature
▽ Transient reduction in lymphocyte count

   The above effects do not appear to be clinically significant

▽ Hypocalcaemia

Drug Interactions

▽ Not to be administered with other biphosphonates or
   mithramycin
▽ Potentiates effect of other hypocalcaemics

Presentation as Aredia

▽ Clear, colourless solution
▽ Ampoules of 15 mg in 5 ml = 3 mg/ml

Dosage as Aredia

Not for direct intravenous injection

Doses of 15 mg, 30 mg, 60 mg or 90 mg are recommended depending on severity of hypercalcaemia

The following rates of infusion are recommended:

15 mg (1 ampoule) in 125 ml 0.9% saline over 2 hours
30 mg (2 ampoules) in 250 ml 0.9% saline over 4 hours
60 mg (4 ampoules) in 500 ml 0.9% saline over 8 hours
90 mg (6 ampoules) in 1 litre 0.9% saline over 24 hours

This should not interfere with mainstay of treatment involving large volumes of intravenous fluids to rehydrate. These infusions should be administered at the above rate concurrently with separate and larger volume infusions to achieve that end

If the drug is to be given by multiple intravenous infusions, the total dose may be given in divided doses over 2–4 days

(e.g.) Total dose of 60 mg may be given as two 30 mg doses mixed as previously described over 2 consecutive days. Therefore, larger volumes of fluid can be administered before and after drug infusion

Effect may be seen at 24–48 hours following administration, maximal at 4–5 days

Monitor electrolyte and calcium responses closely

DISOPYRAMIDE

Proprietary Name

▽ Rythmodan (Roussel Laboratories Ltd)

Indications

▽ Ventricular arrhythmias
▽ Supraventricular arrhythmias } especially post-infarction
▽ Control of venticular and atrial extrasystoles, supraventricular tachycardias and Wolff-Parkinson-White syndrome
▽ Control of arrhythmias following digitalis or similar glycosides

Contraindications and Precautions

▽ Second or third degree heart block and sinus node dysfunction if no pacemaker is present
▽ Hypersensitivity to disopyramide
▽ Cardiogenic shock and severe heart failure
▽ Atrial flutter or tachycardia with block
▽ Caution in glaucoma and prostatism
▽ Reduce dose in renal impairment

Side-effects

▽ Anticholinergic effects
▽ Myocardial depression, hypotension and AV block

Drug Interactions

▽ Amiodarone increases risk of ventricular arrhythmias
▽ Other antiarrhythmics may further depress myocardium
▽ Disopyramide toxicity may be more severe in diuretic-induced hypokalaemia
▽ Rifampicin, phenobarbitone, phenytoin reduce plasma concentration
▽ Anticholinergics may further increase anticholinergic effects

Presentation as Rythmodan

▽ Clear, colourless solution
▽ Ampoule of 50 mg in 5 ml = 10 mg/ml

Dosage as Rythmodan

Infusion should follow initial direct intravenous injections of
2 mg/kg in not less than 5 minutes (to a maximum of 150 mg)
Infusion recommended for patients with serious recurring
arrhythmias being treated in coronary care units or unable
to tolerate oral administration

Rate of 0.4 mg/kg per hour

For a 60 kg adult = 24 mg per hour

Mix 3 × 50 mg ampoules in 500 ml of 0.9% saline or 5% dextrose
Therefore, 150 mg in 500 ml = 0.3 mg/ml

At 24 mg per hour = $24 \times \dfrac{1}{0.3}$ = 80 ml per hour

If less fluid is indicated
Mix 2 × 50 mg ampoules in 100 ml
Therefore, 100 mg in 100 ml
= 1 mg/ml
At 24 mg per hour = 24 ml per hour

Maximum doses recommended are 30 mg per hour
(= 75 kg adult)
30 mg in any one hour
800 mg in any one 24 hour period

DOBUTAMINE HYDROCHLORIDE

Proprietary Name

▽ Dobutrex (Eli Lilly and Co. Ltd)

Indications

▽ Inotropic support in low output cardiac failure associated with myocardial infarction, open heart surgery, cardiomyopathies, septic shock and cardiogenic shock
▽ To maintain cardiac output during PEEP
▽ For cardiac stress testing as an alternative to exercise where exercise is not feasible

Contraindications and Precautions

▽ Hypersensitivity to dobutamine
▽ Pregnancy
▽ Care in recent myocardial infarction
▽ N.B. vital signs and ECG monitoring are essential during therapy

Side-effects

▽ May precipitate or exacerbate ventricular ectopic activity
▽ Rarely has caused ventricular fibrillation or tachycardia
▽ The significant increase in heart rate or arterial pressure may exacerbate ischaemia in acute infarction but has not been shown to increase infarct size
▽ Excessive tachycardia and marked increase in systolic blood pressure in excess dose
▽ Rarely nausea and vomiting
▽ Headache
▽ Palpitations
▽ Hypersensitivity reactions
▽ Phlebitis
▽ Occasionally a precipitous drop in blood pressure has been seen with therapy

Presentation as Dobutrex

▽ Clear, colourless solution
▽ Ampoule of 250 mg in 20 ml = 12.5 mg/ml

Dosage as Dobutrex

Mix 1 ampoule in 500 ml 5% dextrose or 0.9% saline
Therefore, concentration of 500 µg/ml

Infuse at 2.5–10 µg/kg per minute varying according to response
Use IV drip chamber or other monitoring device

Minimum rate for 60 kg adult
2.5 µg × 60 per minute
 = 150 µg per minute
 = 150/500 ml per minute
 = 0.3 ml per minute
 = 0.3 × 60 = 18 ml per hour

Similarly, intermediate rate for 60 kg adult
5 µg × 60 per minute
 = 300 µg per minute
 = 30/500 ml per minute
 = 0.6 ml per minute
 = 0.6 × 60 = 36 ml per hour

Maximum rate for 60 kg adult
10 µg × 60 per minute
 = 600 µg per minute
 = 600/500 ml per minute
 = 1.2 ml per minute
 = 1.2 × 60 = 72 ml per hour

N.B. doses up to 40 µg/kg per minute have been used at the clinician's discretion

If less fluid load is indicated the following regimen may be used

Mix 2 × 250 mg vials (in 40 ml) in 250 ml solution having first removed 40 ml from the bag
Therefore concentration of 2 mg/ml

continued overleaf

Minimum rate for 60 kg adult
2.5 μg × 60 per minute
      = 150 μg per minute
      = 150/2000 ml per minute
      = 0.075 ml/minute
      = 4.5 ml per hour
Intermediate rate for 60 kg adult
5 μg × 60 per minute
      = 300 μg per minute
      = 300/2000 ml per minute
      = 0.15 ml per minute
      = 9 ml per hour

Maximum rate for 60 kg adult
10 μg × 60 per minute
      = 600 μg per minute
      = 600/2000 ml per minute
      = 0.3 ml per minute
      = 18 ml per hour

DOPAMINE HYDROCHLORIDE

Proprietary Name

▽ Dopamine Hydrochloride in 5% Dextrose Injection
(Abbott Laboratories Ltd)
▽ Intropin (Du Pont UK Ltd)

Indications

▽ Cardiogenic shock following infarction especially with
impending renal failure
▽ Cardiac surgery
▽ Endotoxic septicaemia

Contraindications and Precautions

▽ Phaeochromocytoma
▽ Uncorrected tachyarrhythmias or ventricular fibrillation
▽ Care in myocardial infarction
▽ Hypovolaemia should be corrected prior to treatment
▽ Peripheral vascular disease
▽ Care to avoid extravasation at infusion site

Side-effects

▽ Tachycardia and ectopic beats
▽ Anginal pains
▽ Hypotension or hypertension
▽ Peripheral vasoconstriction
▽ Nausea and vomiting

Drug Interactions

▽ Monoamine oxidase inhibitors (MAOIs)
▽ Cyclopropane and halogenated anaesthetics
▽ Inactivated by bicarbonate and other alkaline solutions

Presentation as Dopamine and Intropin

▽ Clear, colourless solution
▽ Ampoule presentation *see* Dosage

Dosage

Preferably via caval catheter

Non-proprietary dopamine hydrochloride

    5 ml ampoule of   40 mg/ml = 200 mg
or 5 ml ampoule of 160 mg/ml = 800 mg

Intropin in similar containers

Mix as 800 mg in 500 ml 0.9% saline or 5% dextrose
Concentration – 1.6 mg/ml = 1600 µg/ml

Infuse at 2–5 µg/kg per minute initially
Adjust dose according to response, for example, to 20 µg/kg
per minute

(e.g.) for 60 kg adult
  2 µg/kg per minute =   2(60 × 60) =   7200 µg per hour =
    4.5 ml per hour
  5 µg/kg per minute =   5(60 × 60) = 18000 µg per hour =
    11.25 ml per hour
10 µg/kg per minute = 10(60 × 60) = 36000 µg per hour =
    22.5 ml per hour
15 µg/kg per minute = 15(60 × 60) = 54000 µg per hour =
    33.75 ml per hour
20 µg/kg per minute = 20(60 × 60) = 72000 µg per hour =
    45 ml per hour

Abbott supply dopamine hydrochloride infusion in 250 ml
5% dextrose at 3 concentrations

    800 µg/ml
    1.6 mg/ml
    3.2 mg/ml

Adjust infusion rate according to concentration

DOXAPRAM HYDROCHLORIDE

Proprietary Name

▽ Dopram (Wyeth Laboratories Ltd)

Indications

▽ To stimulate ventilation in order to avoid using artificial ventilatory support, especially where carbon dioxide retention precludes this management
▽ May also be indicated following anaesthesia

Contraindications and Precautions

▽ Severe hypertension
▽ Status asthmaticus
▽ Coronary artery disease
▽ Thyrotoxicosis
▽ Epilepsy
▽ Physical obstruction of the airway
▽ Pregnancy

Side-effects

▽ Increase in blood pressure
▽ Tachycardia
▽ Dizziness and perineal warmth

Drug Interactions

▽ Theophylline may stimulate CNS
▽ Sympathomimetics potentiate effects on the heart

Presentation as Dopram

▽ Clear, colourless solution
▽ Presented as made up infusion of 1 g in 500 ml
   5% dextrose = 2 mg/ml
▽ Also ampoule 100 mg in 5 ml = 20 mg/ml

Dosage as Dopram

Dose of 1.5–4 mg per minute, adjusted according to response

The manufacturer recommends the following reducing regimen for rapid production of a steady-state plasma concentration

0–15 min 4 mg per min	= 2 ml per min	= 120 ml per hour
13–30 min 3 mg per min	= 1.5 ml per min	= 90 ml per hour
30–60 min 2 mg per min	1 ml per min	= 60 ml per hour
60 min onwards 1.5 mg per min	= 0.75 ml per min	= 45 ml per hour

ERYTHROMYCIN LACTOBIONATE

Proprietary Name

▽ Erythromycin IV lactobionate (Abbott Laboratories Ltd)

Indications

Severe infections caused by sensitive organisms where high blood levels are required at the earliest opportunity or where the oral route is compromised, e.g.

▽ Respiratory tract infections
▽ Skin and soft tissue infections
▽ Gastrointestinal and biliary infections
▽ Endocarditis
▽ Septicaemia
▽ Prophylaxis in surgery, trauma, burns

Contraindications and Precautions

▽ Known hypersensitivity to erythromycin
▽ Impaired hepatic function
▽ Porphyria

Side-effects

▽ Allergy
▽ Gastrointestinal symptoms
▽ Reversible hearing loss in large doses
▽ Reversible cholestatic jaundice

Drug Interactions

May increase plasma concentrations of disopyramide, oral anticoagulants, theophylline, cyclosporin, triazolam, digoxin and carbamazepine

Presentation as Erythromycin IV lactobionate

▽ White powder
▽ Vial of 1 g to be reconstituted and further diluted (may be
  presented with complete drug delivery system)

Dosage as Erythromycin IV lactobionate

Doses up to 50 mg/kg per day in severe infections or the
                immunocompromised
                (e.g.) 60 kg adult = 3 g per day
                25 mg/kg per day in mild to moderate infections
                where oral route is compromised
                (e.g.) 60 kg adult = 1.5 g per day

Infuse either continuously (up to 0.1% solution concentration) or
every 6 hours (up to 0.5% solution) in infusions of 20–60
minutes.

N.B. Higher concentrations may result in pain at infusion site

For example continuous infusion to achieve total dose of 3 g per day

Mix 1 g vial in 1 litre 0.9% saline or 5% glucose (concentration
0.1% i.e. 1 mg/ml) and infuse over 8 hours, repeating three times
in 24 hours

For example intermittent infusion to achieve total dose of 3 g
per day

Mix 750 mg (¾ of vial) in 250 ml 0.9% saline or 5% dextrose
(concentration 0.3% i.e. 3 mg/ml) and infuse over 20–60 minutes
Repeating at 6-hourly intervals

FLECAINIDE

Proprietary Name

▽ Tambocor (3M Riker)

Indications

▽ Ventricular tachycardia (symptomatic, sustained and resistant to other treatment)
▽ Wolff-Parkinson-White syndrome

Contraindications and Precautions

▽ Cardiac failure, asymptomatic non-sustained VT post-infarction
▽ Sinus node dysfunction
▽ Atrial conduction defects
▽ Second degree or greater atrioventricular block
▽ Bundle branch block or distal block
▽ Caution in elderly, reduced hepatic function or renal impairment, patients with pacemakers (can alter thresholds)
▽ Care if electrolytes are deranged

Side-effects

▽ Pro-arrhythmias
▽ Dizziness
▽ Visual disturbances
▽ Nausea and vomiting – rarely

Drug Interactions

▽ Amiodarone increases flecainide concentrations therefore reduce flecainide dose by 50%
▽ Other antiarrhythmic agents increase myocardial depression
▽ Cimetidine increases plasma flecainide concentration
▽ Diuretics – toxicity is increased when hypokalaemia present
▽ Flecainide may increase plasma digoxin levels, although this is unlikely to be of clinical significance

Presentation as Tambocor

▽ Clear, colourless solution
▽ Ampoule of 150 mg in 15 ml = 10 mg/ml

Dosage as Tambocor

Initial bolus injection of 2 mg/kg over not less than 10 minutes
(e.g.) 60 kg adult = 120 mg (maximum for any weight is 150 mg)
Ampoule contains 150 mg in 15 ml. Therefore, use 12 ml
May be added to 100 ml 5% dextrose and infused over 30
minutes
When prolonged parenteral administration is required administer
initial bolus and continue infusion at the following rates
Stop infusion when arrhythmia is controlled

First hour: 1.5 mg/kg per hour
(e.g.) 60 kg adult = 1.5 × 60 = 90 mg per hour
Mix 9 ml of injection in 100 ml 5% dextrose and administer over
one hour

Second and later hours: 0.1–0.25 mg/kg per hour
Add 15 ml of injection to 500 ml 5% dextrose or 0.9% saline
Strength of solution = 0.3 mg/ml
e.g. for 60 kg adult:
Infusion rate: 0.1 mg/kg per hour = 0.1 × 60 = 6 mg per hour
= 6/0.3 ml per hour = 20 ml per hour
0.25 mg/kg per hour = 0.25 × 60 = 15 mg per hour
= 15/0.3 ml per hour = 50 ml per hour
Continuous ECG monitoring is recommended

FLUCYTOSINE

Proprietary Name

▽ Alcobon (Roche Products Ltd)

Indications

▽ Systemic infections with *Cryptococcus* and *Candida* where oral route inappropriate

Contraindications and Precautions

▽ Pregnancy and lactation
▽ Blood dyscrasias
▽ Hepatic and renal impairment

Side-effects

▽ Gastrointestinal symptoms
▽ Rashes
▽ Blood dyscrasias
▽ Changes in liver function tests

Presentation as Alcobon

▽ Colourless to slightly-yellow solution
▽ Infusion bottle containing 2.5 g in 250 ml = 10 mg/ml

Dosage as Alcobon

Dose varies with renal function (*see* data sheet)

The usual dose is 100–200 mg/kg per day in 4 divided doses (e.g. for 60 kg adult)

Minimum dose = 100 × 60 mg per day
⠀⠀⠀⠀⠀⠀⠀⠀⠀ = 6000 mg per day
= 1500 mg qds
150 ml of infusion solution qds over 20–40 minutes

Maximum dose = 200 × 60 mg per day
⠀⠀⠀⠀⠀⠀⠀⠀⠀⠀ = 12,000 mg per day

= 300 mg qds
300 ml (250 ml + 50 ml) of infusion solution qds over 20–40 minutes

FLUMAZENIL

Proprietary Name

▽ Anexate (Roche Products Ltd)

Indications

▽ Complete or partial reversal of the central sedative effects of benzodiazepines. Uses may include reversal of these effects in anaesthesia or in intensive care patients sedated with benzodiazepines

Contraindications and Precautions

▽ Hypersensitivity to benzodiazepines
▽ Epileptics receiving prolonged benzodiazepine treatment (may precipitate convulsions)
▽ Pregnancy
▽ Any patient receiving prolonged benzodiazepine treatment (may precipitate withdrawal symptoms)
▽ Should not be given in anaesthesia reversal until the effects of neuromuscular blockade have cleared
▽ Patients should not drive, operate machinery, etc. for at least 24 hours

Side-effects

▽ Nausea and vomiting
▽ Flushing
▽ Rapid awakening may lead to anxiety and agitation
▽ Transient increases in heart-rate and blood pressure during awakening in intensive care patients
▽ Rarely convulsions (particularly in epileptics)
▽ Rapid injection may precipitate symptoms of benzodiazepine withdrawal

Drug Interactions

▽ Therapeutic action is by way of benzodiazepine antagonism

Presentation as Anexate

▽ Colourless solution
▽ Ampoule of 500 µg in 5 ml = 100 µg/ml

Dosage as Anexate

Administration usually recommended by bolus of 200 µg (2 ml) intravenously over 15 seconds
If desired level of consciousness not obtained, this may be repeated with doses of 100 µg at 60-second intervals where necessary
Maximum recommended dose 1–2 mg
Usual dose required 300–600 µg

Intravenous infusion may be required in recurring drowsiness
Normally a dose of 100–400 µg per hour is used, but the rate should be individually adjusted to achieve the desired level of arousal

Mix 4 ampoules in 500 ml 0.9% saline or 5% glucose
    = 2000 µg in 500 ml
    = concentration of 4 µg/ml

100 µg per hour = 100/4 ml per hour =   25 ml per hour
200 µg per hour = 200/4 ml per hour =   50 ml per hour
300 µg per hour = 300/4 ml per hour =   75 ml per hour
400 µg per hour = 400/4 ml per hour = 100 ml per hour

HEPARIN

Proprietary Name

▽ Monoparin (CP Pharmaceuticals Ltd)
▽ Multiparin (CP Pharmaceuticals Ltd)
▽ Unihep (Leo Laboratories)
▽ Uniparin (CP Pharmaceuticals Ltd)

Indications

▽ Treatment of thrombo-embolic disorders, such as deep vein thrombosis, pulmonary embolism, disseminated intravascular coagulation, fat embolism

Contraindications and Precautions

▽ Haemorrhagic disorders and patients with actual or potential bleeding sites, (e.g.) peptic ulcer
▽ Cerebral aneurysm or recent cerebral haemorrhage
▽ Pregnancy
▽ Severe renal or liver dysfunction
▽ Hypersensitivity
▽ Recent surgery especially of the nervous system or eye
▽ Severe hypertension

Side-effects

▽ Haemorrhage
▽ Hypersensitivity
▽ Thrombocytopenia
▽ Alopecia and osteoporosis (prolonged use)

Drug Interactions

▽ Aspirin and dipyridamole enhance anticoagulant effects

Presentation

▽ Clear, colourless or slightly straw-coloured solutions
▽ Many preparations in different ampoule sizes and
concentrations

Dosage as heparin sodium (non-proprietary), Monoparin, Multiparin, Unihep or Uniparin

Dosage of 20,000–40,000 units per 24 hours

Mix heparin with 0.9% saline or 5% dextrose

Advisable to use portable syringe pump to administer
(e.g.) 20 ml solution over 24 hours

Check therapeutic effect with clotting tests

IMIPENEM WITH CILASTATIN

Proprietary Name

▽ Primaxin (Merck, Sharp and Dohme Ltd)

Indications

▽ Infections caused by susceptible organisms. These include a wide spectrum of Gram-positive, Gram-negative aerobic and anaerobic bacteria. Prophylaxis in certain operative procedures where infection is potentially serious
▽ Not indicated for CNS infections
▽ Due to lack of data, not recommended by manufacturers for use alone in neutropenic patients

Contraindications and Precautions

▽ Hypersensitivity including other beta-lactam antibiotics
▽ Pregnancy and lactation
▽ Children
▽ Renal dysfunction (reduce dose)
▽ CNS disorders, including epilepsy
▽ History of gastrointestinal disease, particularly colitis

Side-effects

▽ Gastrointestinal symptoms, including pseudomembranous colitis
▽ Glossitis and pharyngeal pain (cause unknown)
▽ Blood dyscrasias
▽ Hypersensitivity phenomena
▽ Convulsions, myoclonic activity and confusion
▽ Local thrombophlebitis
▽ Abnormal liver function tests
▽ Renal function: elevated serum creatinine and blood urea have been seen

Drug Interactions

▽ Probenecid decreases excretion

Presentation as Primaxin

▽ White powder
▽ Vials of 250 mg imipenem (with 250 mg cilastatin) and 500 mg
   imipenem (with 500 mg cilastatin) for reconstitution with 50
   and 100 ml solution respectively and direct infusion from vial

Dosage as Primaxin

Recommended dose of 250–500 mg imipenem tds – qds
i.e. 1–2 g Primaxin daily in 3–4 equally divided doses

Doses should be altered depending on renal function and severity
of infection, to a maximum of 50 mg/kg/day or not exceeding
4 g daily

Infuse solution over 20–30 minutes for 250 mg or 500 mg dose
and 40–60 minutes for 1000 mg dose

INSULIN

Indications

▽ Diabetes mellitus and diabetic ketoacidosis

Contraindications and Precautions

▽ Hypoglycaemia
▽ Hypersensitivity
▽ Renal impairment

Side-effects

▽ Overdose causes hypoglycaemia
▽ Hypokalaemia

Drug Interactions

▽ Action antagonized by corticosteroids, diuretics and diazoxide, oral contraceptives, MAOIs
▽ Enhanced by beta-blockers which may mask hypoglycaemic symptoms

Dosage as soluble insulin

Many different preparations and treatment regimens are available

There are various ways of treating ketoacidosis. Rehydration is an extremely important aspect of therapy. Insulin may be administered subcutaneously, intramuscularly or intravenously either continuously or intermittently. Dose depends on blood chemistry which should be regularly monitored and against which the dose should be titrated

A typical regimen may involve two infusions via a single venous line, the first providing fluid (usually in the form of 0.9% saline with or without potassium) and the second, insulin

The soluble insulin may be mixed as 50 units in 50 ml 0.9% saline

Thus corresponding insulin requirement may be as follows:

Blood glucose in mmol per hour	Insulin requirement		
<3.5	½–1 unit per hour	=	½–1 ml per hour
3.5–5	1 unit per hour	=	1 ml per hour
5–7	2 units per hour	=	2 ml per hour
7–11	3 units per hour	=	3 ml per hour
11–14	4 units per hour	=	4 ml per hour
14–18	5 units per hour	=	5 ml per hour
18–22	6 units per hour	=	6 ml per hour
>22	8 units per hour	=	8 ml per hour

It must be emphasized that requirements vary between individual patients and situations

If administration of concentrations such as these via syringe driver or low volume pump is impossible, greater dilutions may be infused with due attention to additional fluid load

ISOPRENALINE HYDROCHLORIDE

Proprietary Name

▽ Saventrine (Pharmax Ltd)

Indications

▽ Cardiogenic or endotoxic shock states
▽ Acute Stokes-Adams attacks and other cardiac emergencies including complete heart block
▽ Severe bradycardia precipitated by beta-adrenergic antagonists and disopyramide
▽ Evaluation of congenital heart defects

Contraindications and Precautions

▽ Acute coronary disease and in patients prone to episodes of ventricular arrhythmias secondary to their slow rate
▽ Care in ischaemic heart disease, diabetes mellitus and hyperthyroidism

Side-effects

▽ Palpitations and precordial pain, tachycardia and hypotension
▽ Tremor and sweats
▽ Facial flushing and headaches

Drug Interactions

▽ May induce arrhythmias when administered with some anaesthetics (namely halothane, cyclopropane, trichloroethylene)

Presentation as Saventrine

▽ Clear, colourless solution
▽ Ampoule of 2 mg in 2 ml = 1 mg/ml

Dosage as Saventrine

Dose of between 0.5 and 10 μg per minute
Severe bradycardias respond to 1–4 μg per minute
Acute Stokes-Adams attacks: 4–8 μg per minute
Shock state: 0.5–10 μg per minute depending on response

Mix in minimum of 500 ml 5% dextrose
Therefore, 1 ampoule = 2000 μg in 500 ml
                    = 4 μg in 1 ml
Therefore, minimum of
  1 μg per minute = 0.25 ml per minute = 15 ml per hour
  5 μg per minute = 1.25 ml   per minute = 75 ml per hour
maximum of
  10 μg per minute = 2.5 ml per minute = 150 ml per hour

ISOSORBIDE DINITRATE AND GLYCERYL TRINITRATE

Proprietary Names

▽ Cedocard (Tillotts Laboratories)
▽ Isoket (Schwarz Pharma Ltd)
▽ Nitrocine (Schwarz Pharma Ltd)
▽ Nitronal (Lipha Pharmaceuticals)
▽ Tridil (Du Pont UK Ltd)

Indications

▽ Unstable angina
▽ Unresponsive cardiac failure
▽ Hypotensive surgery

Contraindications and Precautions

▽ Circulatory collapse, hypotension and cardiogenic shock
▽ Hypersensitivity to nitrates
▽ Uncorrected hypovolaemia
▽ Head trauma or cerebral haemorrhage
▽ Anaemia
▽ Angina caused by hypertrophic obstructive cardiomyopathy (HOCM)
▽ Care in glaucoma
▽ Hypothyroidism
▽ Hypothermia
▽ Severe liver or renal disease
▽ Pregnancy, malnutrition

Side-effects

▽ Hypotension
▽ Headache
▽ Flushing and dizziness
▽ Tachycardia
▽ Nausea
▽ Retrosternal or abdominal discomfort
▽ Restlessness

Drug Interactions

▽ Any drug having an effect on blood pressure will alter effects of nitrates
▽ May also potentiate hypotensive and anticholinergic side-effects of tricyclic antidepressants
▽ May slow the metabolism of morphine-like analgesics

Presentation

▽ *See* Dosage section on next page

Dosage as Isoket or Cedocard

Avoid use with ordinary PVC containers – use polyethylene infusion bags e.g. Polyfusor

Isoket 0.1% is available in ampoules of 10 mg in 10 ml and bottles containing 50 mg in 50 ml and 100 mg in 100 ml
Concentration = 1 mg/ml

Mix 5 ampoules or one 50 ml bottle in 450 ml solution (i.e. 500 ml solution with 50 ml having been removed) = 50 mg in 500 ml

Doses between 2 mg per hour and 10 mg per hour are employed and adjusted according to the response

50 mg in 500 ml = 0.1 mg/ml

Therefore, 2 mg per hour =   20 ml per hour
           5 mg per hour =   50 ml per hour
         10 mg per hour = 100 ml per hour

N.B. If less fluid intake is necessary the infusion rate can be halved by using 100 ml bottle made up to 500 ml with infusion solution. Undiluted 0.05% Isoket may be given via a syringe pump at 500 μg/ml, 4 ml–20 ml per hour

Dosage as Nitrocene, Nitronal or Tridil

3 concentrations are available: use in similar infusion bags to above
5 mg/ml: non-proprietary 25 mg in 5 ml and Tridil 50 mg in 10 ml
1 mg/ml: Nitrocine 10 mg in 10 ml and Nitronal 5 mg in 5 ml, or 50 mg in 50 ml vial
0.5 mg/ml: Tridil 5 mg in 10 ml

Therapeutic dose of 10–200 μg per minute

Therefore, mix 50 mg glyceryl trinitrate in 500 ml infusor = 100 μg/ml

  10 μg per min =   600 μg per hour =   6 ml per hour
  50 μg per min = 3000 μg per hour = 30 ml per hour
100 μg per min = 6000 μg per hour = 60 ml per hour
200 μg per min = 12000 μg per hour = 120 ml per hour

Some preparations are suitable for undiluted administration via a syringe pump if fluid restriction is necessary

ISOXSUPRINE HYDROCHLORIDE

Proprietary Name

▽ Duvadilan (Duphar Laboratories)

Indications

▽ Uncomplicated premature labour

Contraindications and Precautions

▽ Recent arterial haemorrhage
▽ Heart disease
▽ Severe anaemia
▽ Infection
▽ Premature detachment of placenta

Side-effects

▽ Hypotension
▽ Tachycardia
▽ Mild flushing
▽ Nausea and vomiting
▽ Overdose treatment may include use of a non-selective beta-blocker

Presentation

▽ Clear, colourless solution
▽ Ampoule 10 mg in 2 ml = 5mg/ml

Dosage as Duvadilan

Initial dose of 200–300 µg per minute, increased to 500 µg per minute until labour is arrested

Mix 100 mg Duvadilan in 500 ml 5% dextrose or 0.9% saline (or 20 mg Duvadilan in 100 ml 5% dextrose or 0.9% saline) Concentration of 0.2 mg/ml

Rate:

200 µg per minute = 1 ml   per minute =   60 ml per hour
300 µg per minute = 1.5 ml per minute =   90 ml per hour
400 µg per minute = 2 ml   per minute = 120 ml per hour
500 µg per minute = 2.5 ml per minute = 150 ml per hour

N.B. In pregnancy monitoring of vital signs and fluid balance is especially important due to differences in fluid distribution

LABETALOL HYDROCHLORIDE

Proprietary Name

▽ Trandate (Duncan, Flockhart and Co. Ltd)

Indications

▽ Severe hypertension requiring rapid control
▽ Hypertensive episodes following myocardial infarction
▽ Hypertension in pregnancy

Contraindications and Precautions

▽ *See* Atenolol

Side-effects

▽ Excessive postural hypotension may occur if patients are allowed to assume upright position within three hours of dose
▽ Hypersensitivity
▽ Also *see* Atenolol

Drug Interactions

▽ *See* Atenolol

Presentation as Trandate injection

▽ Clear, colourless solution
▽ Ampoule of 100 mg in 20 ml (5 mg/ml)

Dosage as Trandate injection

Single injections of 50 mg (10 ml) can be given over at least one minute. Doses of 50 mg may be repeated at 5 minute intervals until a satisfactory response occurs (maximum total dose of 200 mg)
(Excessive bradycardias can be treated with atropine)

Start infusion at 2 mg per minute (to a maximum of 200 mg) until satisfactory response achieved
Therefore, mix 200 mg (2 ampoules) to 200 ml 5% dextrose or dextrose/saline, concentration = 1 mg/ml

Infuse over 100 minutes at 120 ml per hour
Therefore, 200 mg will be infused over 100 minutes

In hypertension following myocardial infarction
Start at 15 mg per hour, gradually increasing as required to 120 mg per hour
Therefore, mix 200 mg to 200 ml = 1 mg/ml
  15 mg per hour =   15 ml per hour
120 mg per hour = 120 ml per hour

In hypertension of pregnancy
Start at 20 mg per hour, doubled every 30 minutes until control is gained, to a maximum of 160 mg per hour
20 ml per hour to 160 ml per hour with above dilution

LIGNOCAINE HYDROCHLORIDE

Proprietary Name

▽ Xylocard (Astra Pharmaceuticals Ltd)

Indications

▽ Ventricular arrhythmias, especially in recurrent ventricular arrhythmias post-infarction

Contraindications and Precautions

▽ All grades of atrioventricular block
▽ Sino-atrial disorders
▽ Porphyria
▽ Severe myocardial depression
∨ Use with care in cardiac and hepatic failure

Side-effects

▽ Myocardial depression
▽ Dizziness, blurred vision and tremors
▽ Occasionally convulsions and confusion

Drug Interactions

▽ Other cardioactive drugs may increase myocardial depression
▽ Cimetidine inhibits metabolism of lignocaine
▽ Efficacy of lignocaine may be reduced by hypokalaemia following administration of diuretics

Presentation as Xylocard

▽ Clear, colourless solution
▽ Ampoules of 1 g in 5 ml and 2 g in 10 ml = 200 mg/ml

Dosage as Xylocard

Infusion recommended to follow intravenous bolus dose of
50–100 mg. (Approximately 1 mg/kg body weight)
1 g lignocaine in 5 ml = 200 mg/ml
Mix 5 ml ampoule with 1 g into 500 ml 5% dextrose or
0.9% saline

Concentration = 2 mg/ml
Infuse at reducing rates:
First half hour of 4 mg per minute = 2 ml per minute
  = 120 ml per hour
Following two hours at 2 mg per minute = 1 ml per minute
  = 60 ml per hour
Then at 1 mg per minute = ½ ml per minute = 30 ml per hour

METOCLOPRAMIDE HYDROCHLORIDE

Proprietary Name

▽ Maxolon 'High Dose' (Beecham Research)

Indications

▽ Nausea and vomiting as a result of cytotoxic chemotherapy

Contraindications and Precautions

▽ Age—elderly and young (less than 20 years of age)
▽ Renal impairment
▽ Phaeochromocytoma (may precipitate hypertension)
▽ Pregnancy and lactation
▽ Patients receiving other centrally active drugs (e.g. in epilepsy)
▽ Following operations such as pyloroplasty or gut anastomosis (since vigorous muscular contractions may be detrimental to healing)

Side-effects

▽ Extrapyramidal reactions (higher incidence in the younger patient)
▽ Drowsiness, restlessness
▽ Diarrhoea
▽ Hyperprolactinaemia

Drug Interactions

▽ Antagonism by anticholinergics
▽ Absorption of any concurrently administered oral medication may be modified by the effect of metoclopramide on gastric motility
▽ Any drugs causing extrapyramidal side-effects may potentiate those of metoclopramide

Presentation as Maxolon 'High Dose'

▽ Clear, colourless solution
▽ Ampoule of 100 mg in 20 ml = 5 mg/ml

Dosage as Maxolon 'High Dose'

Continuous infusion (recommended method):
Initially (before starting chemotherapy)
2–4 mg/kg over 15–30 minutes in 50–100 ml
(e.g.) 3 × 60 = 180 mg in 100 ml 0.9% saline or 5% dextrose
over 30 minutes

Maintenance dose of 3–5 mg/kg over 8–12 hours in 500 ml
(e.g.) 4 × 60 = 240 mg in 500 ml over 8–12 hours
Total dosage in any 24 hour period should not exceed 10 mg/kg
body-weight

Where cisplatin is to be used the loading dose of Maxolon
'High Dose' should be at least 3 mg/kg body-weight and the
maintenance dose at least 4 mg/kg body-weight

Intermittent infusion (alternative regimen):
Initially (before starting chemotherapy)
Up to 2 mg/kg over at least 15 minutes in at least 50 ml
e.g. 1 × 60 = 60 mg in 50 ml over 15 minutes

Repeat doses of up to 2 mg/kg at 2 hourly intervals in at
least 50 ml
e.g. 1 × 60 = 60 mg in 50 ml over 15 minutes

Total dosage in any 24 hour period should not normally
exceed 10 mg/kg body-weight

METRONIDAZOLE

Proprietary Name

▽ Flagyl (May & Baker Pharmaceuticals)
▽ Zadstat (Lederle Laboratories)

Indications

▽ Prophylaxis and treatment of infections caused by sensitive organisms; active against anaerobic bacteria

Contraindications and Precautions

▽ Hypersensitivity to metronidazole
▽ Disulfiram-like reaction with alcohol
▽ Liver dysfunction
▽ Pregnancy and lactation

Side-effects

▽ Headaches
▽ Rashes
▽ Drowsiness
▽ Dizziness and ataxia
▽ Discoloration of urine
▽ Prolonged therapy may result in neuropathy or seizure

Drug Interactions

▽ Alcohol
▽ Potentiates effect of warfarin
▽ Cimetidine inhibits metabolism
▽ Phenobarbitone accelerates metabolism

Presentation as Flagyl or Zadstat

▽ Clear, colourless solution
▽ Presented as prepared infusion of 500 mg in 100 ml solution

Dosage as Flagyl or Zadstat

Infuse 500 mg 8 hourly over 20 minutes

MEXILETINE HYDROCHLORIDE

Proprietary Name

▽ Mexitil (Boehringer Ingelheim Ltd)

Indications

▽ Existing or anticipated ventricular arrhythmias and ectopics such as occur following infarction or digitalis intoxication

Contraindications and Precautions

▽ High degree of AV block unless pacemaker *in situ*
▽ Cardiogenic shock
▽ Hypersensitivity to mexiletine

Side-effects

▽ Myocardial depression resulting in bradycardia, hypotension, other arrhythmias
▽ Rashes, jaundice and thrombocytopenia
▽ CNS symptoms including confusion, ataxia, convulsions, dysarthria, visual disturbance, tremor and psychosis
▽ Nausea, vomiting and other gastrointestinal disturbances

Drug Interactions

▽ Other cardioactive drugs may potentiate myocardial depression
▽ Rifampicin, phenytoin and phenobarbitone may induce metabolism
▽ Urine acidification or alkalinization may alter elimination

Presentation as Mexitil

▽ Clear, colourless solution
▽ Ampoule of 250 mg in 10 ml = 25 mg/ml

Dosage as Mexitil

Give intravenous loading dose of 4–10 ml (100–250 mg) at 1 ml (25 mg) per minute, i.e. over 4–10 minutes

Then give gradually reducing infusion rate as follows:

Mix 2 ampoules (500 mg) in 500 ml 5% dextrose or 0.9% saline
Concentration = 1 mg/ml

First hour give ∼250 mg = 250 ml
infuse at ∼4 mg/minute = 240 mg per hour
= 240 ml per hour

For second and third hour, infuse remaining ∼250 ml over the two hours, i.e. at 2 mg/minute = 120 ml per hour

The infusion may be reduced to a rate of 0.5 mg per minute = 30 ml per hour

(With the above approximations some solution will remain unused)

Thereafter infuse at 500 µg per minute
Mix one ampoule of 250 mg with 500 ml solution
Concentration = ½ mg/ml = 500 µg per ml
Infuse at 1 ml per minute = 60 ml per hour

MICONAZOLE

Proprietary Name

▽ Daktarin (Janssen Pharmaceuticals Ltd)

Indications

▽ Systemic mycoses including candidosis, aspergillosis and cryptococcosis

Contraindications and Precautions

▽ Hypersensitivity to any of the ingredients
▽ Pregnancy
▽ Porphyria

Side-effects

▽ Local phlebitis
▽ Febrile reactions
▽ Rashes
▽ Gastrointestinal symptoms
▽ Drowsiness
▽ Pruritis
▽ Flushes

Drug Interactions

▽ May potentiate activity of oral anticoagulants, hypoglycaemic agents, phenytoin and other anti-epileptics

Presentation as Daktarin

▽ Clear, colourless solution
▽ Ampoule of 200 mg in 20 ml = 10 mg/ml

Dosage as Daktarin

Recommended adult dose of 600 mg 8 hourly

Mix 3 ampoules in 250–500 ml 0.9% saline or 5% dextrose

Infuse over at least 30 minutes
(more rapid injection may lead to cardiac arrhythmias)

Using a subclavian catheter or changing sites of infusion every 48–72 hours reduces incidence and severity of phlebitis

NAFTIDROFURYL OXALATE

Proprietary Name

▽ Praxilene Forte (Lipha Pharmaceuticals Ltd)

Indications

▽ Acute symptoms of severe peripheral vascular disease

Contraindications and Precautions

▽ Hypersensitivity to naftidrofuryl oxalate
▽ Atrioventricular block
▽ Severe cardiac disease especially with conduction disorders
▽ Renal dysfunction
▽ Hepatic dysfunction
▽ Pregnancy

Side-effects

▽ Nausea
▽ Cardiac block and convulsions in overdose
▽ Epigastric pain

Drug Interactions

▽ Drugs with cardiac actions may have additive effects when used
with naftidrofuryl

Presentation as Praxilene Forte

▽ Clear, colourless solution
▽ Ampoule of 200 mg in 10 ml = 20 mg/ml

Dosage as Praxilene Forte

Must not be given by bolus injection

Recommended dose of 200 mg bd

Mix one ampoule in 250–500 ml 0.9% saline, 5% dextrose or low molecular weight dextran

Infuse over minimum of 90 minutes (e.g.) one ampoule in 250 ml over 2 hours

i.e. 125 ml per hour

NALOXONE

Proprietary Name

▽ Narcan (Du Pont UK Ltd)

Indications

▽ Reversal of opioid depression
▽ Diagnosis of suspected acute opioid overdose

Contraindications and Precautions

▽ Hypersensitivity
▽ Care in opioid dependence (may precipitate acute withdrawal syndrome)

Side-effects

▽ Possible nausea and vomiting – mainly associated with long-term oral administration

Presentation as Narcan

▽ Clear, colourless solution
▽ *See* Dosage section below

Dosage (non-proprietary) or as Narcan

May be given as single injections
Ampoule of 1 ml (400 µg) or 10 ml (4 mg). Also 2 ml (2 mg)
Dilute in 0.9% saline or 5% dextrose to a concentration of
4 µg/ml

(e.g.) Infuse 2 mg in 500 ml
Rate of infusion is response dependent

N.B. Half-life of naloxone may necessitate repeated injections
or infusion as the effect wears off

OXYTOCIN

Proprietary Name

▽ Syntocinon (Sandoz Pharmaceuticals)

Indications

▽ Induction of labour
▽ Stimulation of labour in hypotonic uterine inertia
▽ Management of missed or incomplete abortion
▽ Postpartum haemorrhage in the occasional patient not responding to ergometrine

Contraindications and Precautions

▽ Hypertonic uterine inertia
▽ Mechanical obstruction to delivery
▽ Failed trial of labour
▽ Severe toxaemia
▽ Placenta praevia
▽ Foetal distress
▽ Predisposition to amniotic fluid embolism
▽ Care in abnormal foetal presentation, multiple pregnancy, previous caesarian section, high parity, hypertension
▽ In patients with cardiovascular disorders, infusion volumes must be kept low

Side-effects

▽ Very high doses may cause violent uterine spasm leading to uterine rupture, tissue damage and foetal asphyxiation
▽ Maternal hypertension and subarachnoid haemorrhage

Presentation as Syntocinon

▽ Ampoule of 2 units in 2 ml (1 unit/ml)
                    5 units in 1 ml (5 units/ml)
                    10 units in 1 ml (10 units/ml)
                    50 units in 5 ml (10 units/ml)

Dosage as Syntocinon

Induction and augmentation of labour

Mix 20 units of Syntocinon in 1 litre 5% dextrose or 0.9% saline
Therefore, 50 ml contains 1 unit

Start infusion at 2 mU per minute
             = 120 mU per hour
             = 0.12 units per hour

Adjust according to response

  2 mU per minute = 0.12 units per hour
  = 6 ml per hour
  4 mU per minute = 0.24 units per hour
  = 12 ml per hour
  8 mU per minute = 0.48 units per hour
  = 24 ml per hour
16 mU per minute = 0.96 units per hour
  = 48 ml per hour

Missed abortion

Mix 20 units of Syntocinon in 500 ml 5% dextrose or 0.9% saline

Start infusion at 10 drops per minute = 30 ml per hour
Increase to 90 ml per hour after one hour
Following this doses may be increased every hour to a maximum
of 250 ml per hour
(at maximum dose consider increasing concentration and
therefore reducing fluid load)

Postpartum haemorrhage

Mix 10 units Syntocinon in 500 ml of fluid
Give 15 drops per minute = 45 ml per hour
Adjust according to response

POLYMYXIN B SULPHATE

Proprietary Name

▽ Aerosporin (Calmic Medical Division)

Indications

▽ An alternative antibacterial therapy in severe systemic Gram-negative infections including *Pseudomonas*, *E. coli*

Contraindications and Precautions

▽ Hypersensitivity
▽ Renal impairment
▽ Myasthenia gravis

Side-effects

▽ Nephrotoxicity
▽ Circumoral and peripheral paraesthesiae
▽ Vertigo
▽ Muscle weakness
▽ Apnoea
▽ Electrolyte disturbance

Drug Interactions

▽ Muscle relaxants
▽ General anaesthesia
▽ Other antibiotics with muscle relaxant properties

Presentation as Aerosporin

▽ Powder
▽ Ampoule of 500,000 units for reconstitution

Dosage as Aerosporin

Dose of 15,000–25,000 units/kg daily
(e.g.) 20,000 × 60 = 1,200,000 (1.2 M) in 24 hours

Give as continuous infusion or 600,000 units bd
(12 hours apart)
Mix in 500 ml 5% dextrose and infuse over 1–2 hours

N.B. Reduce dose in renal impairment (*see* data sheet)

POTASSIUM CHLORIDE

Indications

▽ Hypokalaemia where enteral route is not possible or where clinical condition requires immediate replacement
▽ Prophylaxis in circumstances where hypokalaemia is likely, e.g. use of insulin in correction of diabetic ketoacidosis

Contraindications and Precautions

▽ *See* Dosage

Side-effects

▽ Rapid administration may cause cardiac arrhythmias or arrest
▽ Overdose may result in hyperkalaemia

Presentation

▽ *See* Dosage section below

Dosage and Administration

Ampoule of 20 mmol KCl in 10 ml, not for direct intravenous injection

0.9% saline and 5% dextrose infusion solutions are supplied with added KCl of 20 mmol per litre in 1 litre bags

If high concentrations of KCl are required, it is recommended that one of two methods be employed, resulting in maximum concentration of 40 mmol KCl per litre:

The addition of a single 10 ml (20 mmol) ampoule to 1 litre of solution already containing 20 mmol KCl
concentration = 40 mmol KCl per litre

The addition of a single 10 ml (20 mmol) ampoule to a 500 ml solution containing no potassium
concentration = 20 mmol KCl in 500 ml
                        (40 mmol KCl per litre)

Any added injection must be mixed thoroughly
The 'normal' blood value of potassium is approximately 3.5–5 mmol per litre

In conditions where rapid administration is required for low blood potassium the following regimen is suggested:

500 ml infusion solution + 20 mmol KCl over 2 hours
or 1 litre infusion solution + 40 mmol KCl over 4 hours
i.e. maximum of equivalent of 10 mmol KCl per hour
Repeat until correction of blood chemistry is achieved

Patient fluid requirements must be closely monitored

Certain clinical occasions may require higher doses of KCl at the discretion of the clinician. Here it is recommended the infusions are pump-controlled, blood electrolytes are regularly monitored and ECG monitoring is available

PROCAINAMIDE HYDROCHLORIDE

Proprietary Name

▽ Pronestyl (Bristol-Myers Squibb Pharmaceuticals Ltd)

Indications

▽ Treatment of symptomatic or potentially malignant ventricular arrhythmias
▽ Especially following myocardial infarction

Contraindications and Precautions

▽ Torsades de pointes
▽ Hypersensitivity to procainamide or related drugs
▽ Myasthenia gravis
▽ High degree of complete AV block, hypotension, asthma
▽ Elderly
▽ Pregnancy
▽ Children
▽ Renal or hepatic dysfunction
▽ Digitalis intoxication
▽ Congestive heart failure
▽ Acute ischaemic heart disease, cardiogenic shock and cardiomyopathy

Side-effects

▽ Hypotension, myocardial depression and cardiac failure
▽ Gastrointestinal symptoms
▽ Allergic phenomena including fever, rashes and pruritis
▽ SLE-like syndrome
▽ Agranulocytosis (after prolonged therapy)

Drug Interactions

▽ Other antiarrhythmics may potentiate myocardial depression
▽ Amiodarone and cimetidine increase plasma procainamide levels

Presentation as Pronestyl

▽ Clear, colourless solution
▽ Vial of 1 g in 10 ml = 100 mg/ml

Dosage as Pronestyl

Administration should be under continuous ECG monitoring

A therapeutic plasma concentration is usually achieved once a dose of 500 to 600 mg has been given over 30 minutes
Thus, mix 600 mg (6 ml of ampoule) in 100 ml 5% dextrose

Alternatively 100 mg bolus injections may be given over a minimum of two minutes at intervals of five minutes until arrhythmias controlled (maximum 1 g) i.e. at a rate no greater than 50 mg per minute
Each 100 mg bolus (1 ml) should be diluted with 5% dextrose for injection in order to facilitate rate of administration

If hypotension occurs rate of administration should be slowed or stopped. Reversal may be achieved by noradrenaline. BP must be closely monitored

Maintenance infusion rate is 2–6 mg per minute

Suggested regimen:

Mix 2 g in 500 ml 5% dextrose (two 10 ml ampoules)

2000 mg in 500 ml = 4 mg/ml

Minimum rate of 2 mg/minute = 0.5 ml/minute = 30 ml/hour
Medium rate of 4 mg/minute = 1 ml/minute = 60 ml/hour
Maximum rate of 6 mg/minute = 1.5 ml/minute = 90 ml/hour

QUININE DIHYDROCHLORIDE

Indications

▽ Falciparum malaria

Contraindications and Precautions

▽ Cardiac conduction defects
▽ Atrial fibrillation
▽ Pregnancy
▽ Haemoglobinuria
▽ Optic neuritis

Side-effects

▽ Chinchonism (headache, gastrointestinal symptoms, tinnitus, confusion and rashes)
▽ Hypersensitivity

Drug Interactions

▽ Cardiac glycosides (plasma concentrations of digoxin increased)
▽ Cimetidine inhibits metabolism

Presentation

▽ *See* Dosage section below

Dosage

Ampoule of 300 mg/ml in 1 ml (300 mg) or 2 ml (600 mg)

Loading dose of 20 mg/kg in 4 hours

20 mg × 60 kg = 1200 mg
(e.g. mix 4 × 1 ml or 2 × 2 ml ampoule in 500 ml 0.9% saline)
Infuse 500 ml in 4 hours

Maintenance dose of
  10 mg/kg in 4 hours, given 8 hourly
  e.g. 10 × 60 = 600 mg
Infuse in 250–500 ml 0.9% saline in 4 hours

RIFAMPICIN

Proprietary Names

▽ Rifadin (Merrell Dow Pharmaceuticals Ltd)
▽ Rimactane (Ciba Laboratories)

Indications

▽ Tuberculosis infection where oral route inappropriate

Contraindications and Precautions

▽ Hypersensitivity to rifamycins
▽ Pregnancy
▽ Impaired liver function
▽ Elderly and children
▽ Porphyria

Side-effects

▽ Hypersensitivity including rashes and fever
▽ Flushing and itching
▽ Gastrointestinal symptoms
▽ Hepatitis
▽ Thrombocytopenia
▽ 'Flu syndrome' possibly associated with haemolysis, acute renal
  failure and hypotension
▽ Reddish discoloration of body fluids

Drug Interactions

▽ Rifampicin may reduce the activity of the following drugs by
  enzyme induction: oral anticoagulants, corticosteroids,
  cyclosporin, digoxin, oral contraceptives, oral hypoglycaemic
  agents, dapsone, phenytoin, quinidine, narcotics and analgesics,
  propranolol, verapamil and disopyramide, theophylline,
  thyroxine, cimetidine, azathioprine

This list may not be exhaustive

Presentation as Rifadin and Rimactane

▽ Red lyophilized powder
▽ Vials of 600 mg with 10 ml solution and 300 mg with
  5 ml solution for reconstitution

Dosage as Rifadin or Rimactane

Dosage of 600 mg or approximately 10 mg/kg body-weight per day
Following reconstitution dilute in 250 ml (300 mg) or 500 ml
(600 mg) 5% dextrose or 0.9% saline and infuse over 2–3 hours
(not more than 6 hours)

RITODRINE HYDROCHLORIDE

Proprietary Name

▽ Yutopar (Duphar Laboratories Ltd)

Indications

▽ Uncomplicated pre-term labour
▽ Fetal asphyxia in labour where it is desired to obtain uterine relaxation

Contraindications and Precautions

▽ Antepartum haemorrhage which demands immediate delivery
▽ Eclampsia and severe pre-eclampsia
▽ Intra-uterine foetal death
▽ Chorioamnionitis
▽ Maternal cardiac disease and hypertension
▽ Cord compression
▽ Hyperthyroidism
▽ Insulin dependent diabetes mellitus – monitor blood glucose

Side-effects

▽ Tachycardia (aim to maintain heart rate below 140 beats per minute)
▽ Flushing
▽ Pulmonary oedema reported in association with patients treated with corticosteroids and betamimetics
▽ Sweating
▽ Tremor
▽ Nausea and vomiting
▽ Hypokalaemia

Effects of overdose may be reversed by using a nonselective beta-blocker

Drug Interactions

▽ MAOIs
▽ Tricyclic antidepressants
▽ Corticosteroids
▽ Sympathomimetic amines
▽ Anaesthetics
▽ Beta-blockers
▽ Potassium depleting diuretics

Presentation as Yutopar

▽ Clear, colourless solution
▽ Ampoule of 50 mg in 5 ml = 10 mg/ml

Dosage as Yutopar

Mix 100 mg in 500 ml 0.9% saline or 5% dextrose = 0.2 mg/ml
Infuse at 50 µg per minute and increase up to 350 µg per minute

50 µg per minute = 3000 µg per hour = 3000/200 ml per hour
= 15 ml per hour
100 µg per minute = 6000 µg per hour = 6000/200 ml per hour
= 30 ml per hour
200 µg per minute = 12000 µg per hour = 12000/200 ml per hour
- 60 ml per hour
300 µg per minute = 18000 µg per hour = 18000/200 ml per hour
= 90 ml per hour
350 µg per minute = 21000 µg per hour = 21000/200 ml per hour
= 105 ml per hour

An alternative method is to use an infusion pump with 150 mg
ritodrine (3 ampoules) made up to 50 ml with infusion fluid
= 3 mg/ml

50 µg per minute = 3 mg per hour = 1 ml per hour
100 µg per minute = 6 mg per hour = 2 ml per hour
200 µg per minute = 12 mg per hour = 4 ml per hour
300 µg per minute = 18 mg per hour = 6 ml per hour
350 µg per minute = 21 mg per hour = 7 ml per hour

The above regimen is useful when fluid load is to be restricted

Monitoring of vital signs and fluid balance should be performed

SALBUTAMOL AND TERBUTALINE SULPHATE

Proprietary Names

▽ Salbuvent (Tillotts Laboratories)
▽ Ventolin (Allen and Hanburys Ltd)
▽ Bricanyl (Astra Pharmaceuticals)

Indications

▽ For the relief of the bronchospasm of asthma or bronchitis and in status asthmaticus
▽ In the management of uncomplicated premature labour in the last trimester (excluding cases of placenta praevia, toxaemia or antepartum haemorrhage)

Contraindications and Precautions

▽ Hypersensitivity to the drug or infusion components
▽ Threatened abortion in first or second trimester
▽ Care in tachycardias, hypertension and ischaemic heart disease, where positive chronotropic effects of the drug may be harmful
▽ Hyperthyroidism
▽ Diabetes mellitus (likely to increase blood glucose)

Side-effects

▽ Tachycardia
▽ Hypersensitivity reactions
▽ Tremor
▽ Anxiety
▽ Headache
▽ Hypokalaemia and hyperglycaemia
▽ Transient muscle cramps

Drug Interactions

▽ Non-selective beta-blockers
▽ High dose corticosteroids may potentiate hypokalaemia and
   hyperglycaemia

Presentation

▽ *See* Dosage section below

Dosage of salbutamol as Salbuvent or Ventolin solution for intravenous infusion

5 ml ampoule of 1 mg/ml = 5 mg

Mix in 500 ml of 0.9% saline or 5% dextrose (the former may be advisable in diabetics)

For asthma, infuse initially at 5 µg per minute
adjust according to response to a range of 3–20 µg per min
5 mg in 500 ml = 10 µg/ml

```
 3 µg per min = 0.3 ml per min =  18 ml per hour
 5 µg per min = 0.5 ml per min =  30 ml per hour
10 µg per min = 1   ml per min =  60 ml per hour
15 µg per min = 1.5 ml per min =  90 ml per hour
20 µg per min = 2   ml per min = 120 ml per hour
```

To prevent contractions, doses of 10–45 µg per minute are generally adequate, but may need to be altered according to strength and frequency of contractions. Monitor maternal heart rate carefully

It is recommended that the starting dose be 10 µg per minute and increased by units of e.g. 5 µg per minute every 10 minutes until patient responds, unless side-effects preclude such a rapid rise in dose e.g. heart rate > 140 beats per minute. Once contractions have ceased maintain dose for at least 1 hour reducing thereafter by 50% decrements at 6-hourly intervals

Dosage of terbutaline as Bricanyl

Ampoule of 500 µg/ml

1 ml ampoule contains 500 µg
5 ml ampoule contains 2.5 mg

Mix 5 ml ampoule in 500 ml 0.9% saline or 5% dextrose
Therefore, 2.5 mg in 500 ml
2500/500 ml = concentration of 5 µg/ml

continued overleaf

Run at 1.5–5 µg per minute for 8–10 hours

1.5 µg per min =	90 µg per hour =	18 ml per hour
2 µg per min =	120 µg per hour =	24 ml per hour
2.5 µg per min =	150 µg per hour =	30 ml per hour
3 µg per min =	180 µg per hour =	36 ml per hour
3.5 µg per min =	210 µg per hour =	42 ml per hour
4 µg per min =	240 µg per hour =	48 ml per hour
4.5 µg per min =	270 µg per hour =	54 ml per hour
5 µg per min =	300 µg per hour =	60 ml per hour

To prevent contractions: 10 µg per minute initially, increasing by 5 µg per minute at 10 minute intervals until contractions stop, to 25 µg per minute, then reducing to a minimal dose preventing contractions. Monitor maternal heart rate carefully

SODIUM FUSIDATE

Proprietary Name

▽ Fucidin (Leo Laboratories)

Indications

▽ Staphylococcal infections such as osteomyelitis, pneumonia, septicaemia, endocarditis and superinfected cystic fibrosis

Contraindications and Precautions

▽ Hypersensitivity
▽ Liver dysfunction

Side-effects

▽ Nausea and vomiting
▽ Rashes
▽ Reversible jaundice

Presentation as Fucidin

▽ Dry powder
▽ Vial of 500 mg powder to be reconstituted with 50 ml buffer
  supplied

Dosage as Fucidin

Dose of 500 mg tds
Dilute to a maximum of 1 mg/ml with 0.9% saline or
5% dextrose
Infuse over 6 hours

i.e. 500 mg in 500 ml over 6 hours
(minimum dilution and infusion rates)

SODIUM NITROPRUSSIDE

Proprietary Name

▽ Nipride (Roche Products Ltd)

Indications

▽ To reduce blood pressure in hypertensive crisis
▽ To achieve hypotension in surgical procedures
▽ To improve cardiac function in acute or chronic heart failure

Contraindications and Precautions

▽ Compensatory hypertension, e.g. in coarctation of the aorta
▽ Severe hepatic impairment
▽ Vitamin B_{12} deficiency
▽ Leber's optic atrophy
▽ Care in elderly patients and renal impairment
▽ Cerebrovascular disease
▽ Hypothyroidism

Side-effects

▽ Nausea
▽ Apprehension, headache and restlessness, muscle twitching
▽ Retrosternal pain and palpitations
▽ Dizziness and abdominal pain
▽ Precipitous drop in blood pressure

All noted with excessively rapid reduction in blood pressure

▽ Rebound hypertension on sudden withdrawal
▽ Methaemoglobinaemia of cyanide toxicity

Presentation as Nipride

▽ Dry powder
▽ Ampoule of 50 mg to reconstitute with 2 ml solution
  = 25 mg/ml

Dosage as Nipride

Control flow rate with care
Avoid sudden increases or decreases in dose

Dose in hypertensive crisis
Initially 0.3–1 µg/kg per minute
Adjusted as required to 0.5–6 µg/kg per minute depending
on response
Maximum recommended short-term dose is 8 µg/kg per minute

Dose in cardiac failure
Initially 10–15 µg per minute
Increasing every 5–10 minutes by increments of 10–15 µg
per minute
Usual range of 10–200 µg per minute
Maximum 280 µg per minute (4 µg/kg per minute)

Mix 50 mg ampoule in 500 ml 5% dextrose
Therefore, 50 mg in 500 ml
Concentration of 100 µg per ml

Flow rate (µg/kg per minute)	Flow rate for 60 kg adult (µg per minute)	µg per hour	ml per hour
0.3	18	1080	10.8
0.5	30	1800	18
1	60	3600	36
2	120	7200	72
3	180	10800	108
4	240	14400	144
5	300	18000	180
6	360	21600	216

N.B. In high doses, higher concentrations of the infusion mixture
may be needed to prevent fluid overload

SODIUM VALPROATE

Proprietary Name

▽ Epilim (Sanofi UK Ltd)

Indications

▽ Epilepsy

Contraindications and Precautions

▽ Active liver disease or liver dysfunction
▽ Children
▽ Pregnancy, lactation
▽ Diabetics: may give false positive ketonuria results

Side-effects

▽ Liver dysfunction
▽ Gastrointestinal symptoms
▽ Weight gain
▽ Oedema
▽ Transient hair loss
▽ Reversible platelet dysfunction
▽ Hyperammonaemia
▽ Rarely pancreatitis, ataxia, sedation, rashes, amenorrhoea
▽ Mainly associated with long-term oral administration

Drug Interactions

▽ Antidepressants may be potentiated and convulsions more likely
▽ Antipyschotics may lower convulsive threshold (this is a
   property of the antipsychotics themselves)
▽ Aspirin and other anticoagulants may add to possible effects on
   platelet function
▽ Enzyme-inducing drugs including anti-epileptics may reduce
   valproate levels and valproate may itself affect levels of other
   anti-epileptics

Presentation as Epilim

▽ Off-white powder
▽ Vial of 400 mg to be reconstituted with 4 ml solution
    = 100 mg/ml

Dosage as Epilim

Where oral route is temporarily not possible, continue same dose as oral
(e.g.) 600–800 mg tds
Mix appropriate amount in, for example, 250–500 ml 0.9% saline or 5% dextrose and infuse over 1–4 hours

If commencing valproate, slow intravenous injection over 3–5 minutes of 400–800 mg (up to 10 mg/kg) may be used
Then infuse intermittently as above or infuse continuously up to 2500 mg per day
(e.g.) 800 mg in 500 ml over 8 hours
repeated continuously

STREPTOKINASE

Proprietary Names

▽ Kabikinase (KabiVitrum Ltd)
▽ Streptase (Hoechst Ltd)

Indications

▽ Myocardial infarction
▽ Deep vein thrombosis
▽ Acute major pulmonary embolus
▽ Acute arterial thromboembolism
▽ Clearance of clotted haemodialysis shunts

Contraindications and Precautions

▽ Recent surgery or invasive procedures
▽ Recent gastrointestinal bleeding
▽ Thrombocytopenia or evidence of defective haemostasis
▽ Liver or kidney disease
▽ CVA
▽ Severe treated or untreated hypertension
▽ Recent parturition
▽ Ulcerative colitis
▽ Visceral carcinoma
▽ Menstrual bleeding
▽ Pregnancy
▽ Previous exposure to streptokinase or previous hypersensitivity to streptokinase
▽ Current or recent anticoagulation
▽ Recent streptococcal infection
▽ Severe bronchitis, active TB and pneumothorax
▽ Diabetic retinopathy
▽ Potential for cardiac thromboemboli (e.g. active or recent infective endocarditis)

Side-effects

▽ Pyrexia, allergic reactions
▽ Rarely anaphylaxis
▽ Haemorrhage
▽ Arrhythmias, transient hypotension

Drug Interactions

▽ Any drug affecting coagulation will affect pharmacodynamics

N.B. It is recommended that heparinization and oral anticoagulation follow discontinuation of streptokinase to prevent reformation of thrombus, and oral aspirin following myocardial infaction for at least 4 weeks

▽ Administration of corticosteroid with streptokinase should be considered to avoid allergic reactions
▽ Haemorrhage may be reversed by tranexamic acid 10 mg/kg by slow intravenous injection

Presentation as Kabikinase or Streptase

▽ Straw-coloured lyophilized powder
▽ Available in vials of 100,000, 250,000, 600,000, 750,000
and 1,500,000 units for reconstitution

Dosage as Kabikinase or Streptase

Dose in myocardial infarction
1,500,000 (1.5 million units) in 100 ml 0.9% saline or 5% dextrose
infused over 60 minutes

Dose in deep vein thrombosis, pulmonary embolism or arterial
thrombosis
Load with 250,000 to 600,000 units over 30 minutes
Then maintenance dose of 100,000 units per hour for
24–72 hours (depending on condition)
(e.g.) Mix 1,000,000 (1 million units) in 500 ml 0.9% saline or
5% dextrose and infuse over 10 hours

In view of continuing research, please refer to manufacturers'
information for latest full data sheets

TETRACYCLINE HYDROCHLORIDE

Proprietary Name

▽ Achromycin (Lederle Laboratories)

Indications

▽ Infections caused by sensitive organisms, which include *Borrellia, Calymmatobacterium, Chlamydia, Haemophilus, Mycoplasma* and *Rickettsia* species
▽ Also infections due to *Listeria, Bordetella, Treponema, Neisseria* and *Shigella*

Contraindications and Precautions

▽ Hypersensitivity to tetracyclines
∨ Renal failure
▽ Pregnancy and lactation
▽ Children under 12 years
▽ SLE
▽ Hepatic insufficiency

Side-effects

▽ Gastrointestinal symptoms
▽ Hypersensitivity
▽ Overgrowth of resistant or non-susceptible organisms
▽ Uraemia, hyperphosphataemia and acidosis due to accumulation in renal failure
▽ Raised intracranial pressure and enamel hypoplasia in infants (contraindicated)

Drug Interactions

▽ Methoxyflurane anaesthetic increases risk of renal failure
▽ Potentiates effect of anticoagulants

Presentation as Achromycin

▽ Yellow powder
▽ Vials of 250 mg or 500 mg to be reconstituted with 5 or 10 ml solution respectively

Dosage as Achromycin

Recommended dose of 500 mg twice a day (to maximum of 2 g daily)

Mix 500 mg tetracycline in 250–500 ml 0.9% saline or 5% dextrose
Infuse solution over 1–3 hours
i.e. in 100–1000 ml solution at a rate not exceeding 100 ml in 5 minutes

Infusion should be immediately following reconstitution and dilution

THEOPHYLLINE AND AMINOPHYLLINE

Proprietary Name

▽ Labophylline (Laboratories for Applied Biology Ltd)

Indications

▽ Reversible airways obstruction including acute asthma

Contraindications and Precautions

▽ Known hypersensitivity to xanthine preparations
▽ Care in patients previously receiving oral xanthines
▽ Elderly
▽ Lactation
▽ Cardiac disease
▽ Liver disease
▽ Epilepsy
▽ Concurrent viral infections with pyrexia

Side-effects

▽ Tachycardia and palpitations
▽ Arrhythmias
▽ Convulsions
▽ Gastrointestinal disturbances

Drug Interactions

▽ Plasma concentrations are affected by: antiepileptics, including
barbiturates, oral contraceptive pill, antibiotics, including
erythromycin and ciprofloxacin, calcium-channel blockers
including verapamil, cimetidine, sulphinpyrazone, rifampicin
▽ Theophyllines may affect plasma lithium levels

Presentation as Labophylline

▽ *See* Dosage section below

Dosage as aminophylline (ethylene-diamine theophylline)

If not already taking oral xanthines
Loading dose of 250–500 mg (5 mg/kg)
over 20 minutes e.g. mixed with 100 ml 0.9% saline
Followed by maintenance infusion at 500 µg/kg per hour

Ampoule contains 250 mg in 10 ml
Mix 250 mg in 500 ml 0.9% saline or 5% dextrose
Therefore, concentration of 500 µg/ml
(e.g.) for 60 kg adult
500 µg × 60 per hour
= 1 ml solution × 60 per hour
= 60 ml per hour
i.e. 1 ml/kg

Dosage as Labophylline (lysine theophylline)

Slow injection of 200 mg over 20 minutes
Followed by infusion at a rate of 500 µg/kg per hour

1 ampoule contains 200 mg in 10 ml

Mix 200 mg in 500 ml 0.9% saline or 5% dextrose
Concentration = 400 µg/ml

(e.g.) for 60 kg adult
500 µg × 60 per hour = 30,000 µg per hour
30,000/400 = 75 ml per hour
After 12 hours reduce to 400 µg/kg per hour = 60 ml per hour

It may be inadvisable to give the above doses to patients who
have taken theophylline within the last 24 hours. Where
clinically necessary the dose may be reduced but risk of xanthine
toxicity must be carefully considered.

APPENDIX 1

Poisons Information Services

Belfast	0232 240503

Birmingham	021 554 3801

Cardiff	0222 709901

Dublin	0001 379964/379966

Edinburgh	031 229 2477/228 2441 (Viewdata)

Leeds	0532 430715/432799

London	071 635 9191/955 5000

Newcastle	091 232 5131

Some of these centres also advise on analysis services offered by laboratories which may help in the diagnosis and management of some cases.

APPENDIX 2

Addresses of pharmaceutical companies

3M Riker
3M House
Morley Street
Loughborough
Leicestershire
LE11 1EP
0509 611611

Abbott Laboratories Ltd
Abbott House
Moorbridge Road
Maidenhead
Berkshire
SL6 8JG
0628 773355

Allen & Hanburys Ltd
2 Ironbridge Road
Stockley Park
Uxbridge
Middlesex
UB11 1BT
081 422 4225

Astra Pharmaceuticals
Home Park Estate
Kings Langley
Herts
WD4 8DH
09277 66191

Boehringer Ingelheim Ltd
Ellesfield Avenue
Bracknell
Berkshire
RG12 4YS
0344 424600

Bristol-Myers Squibb Pharmaceuticals Ltd
Squibb House
141/149 Staines Road
Hounslow
TW3 3JA
081 572 7422

Calmic Medical Division
see Wellcome Medical Division

Ciba Laboratories
Wimblehurst Road
Horsham
West Sussex
RH12 4AB
0403 50101

CP Pharmaceuticals Ltd
Ash Road North
Wrexham Industrial Estate
Wrexham
Clwyd
LL13 9UF
0978 661261

Dumex Pharmaceuticals
Longwick Road
Princes Risborough
Aylesbury
Bucks
HP17 9UZ
0844 274414

Duncan Flockhart & Co Ltd
Horsenden House
Greenford Road
Greenford
Middlesex
UB6 0HE
081 422 3434

Duphar Laboratories Ltd
Gaters Hill
West End
Southampton
SO3 3JD
0703 472281

Du Pont UK Ltd
Wedgwood Way
Stevenage
Hertfordshire
SG1 4QN
0438 734550

Eli Lilly & Co Ltd
Kingsclere Road
Basingstoke
Hampshire
RG21 2XA
0256 473241

Farmitalia Carlo Erba Ltd
Italia House
23 Grosvenor Road
St Albans
AL1 3AW
0727 40041

Glaxo Pharmaceuticals UK Ltd
891/995 Greenford Road
Greenford
Middlesex
UB6 0HE
081 422 3434

Hoechst UK Ltd
Hoechst House
Salisbury Road
Hounslow
Middlesex
TW4 6JH
081 570 7712

Janssen Pharmaceutical Ltd
Grove
Wantage
Oxon
OX12 0DQ
0235 772966

KabiVitrum Ltd
3 Dukes Meadow
Millboard Road
Bourne End
Bucks
SL8 5XF
0628 850300

Laboratories for Applied Biology Ltd
91 Amhurst Park
London
N16 5DR
081 800 2252

Lederle Laboratories
154 Fareham Road
Gosport
Hants
PO13 0AS
0329 224000

Leo Laboratories Ltd
Longwick Road
Princes Risborough
Aylesbury
Bucks
HP17 9RR
08444 7333

Lipha Pharmaceuticals Ltd
Harrier House
High Street
West Drayton
Middlesex
UB7 7QG
0895 449331

May & Baker Pharmaceuticals
Rhône–Poulenc UK Ltd
Rainham Road South
Dagenham
Essex
RM10 7XS
081 592 3060

Merck Sharp & Dohme Ltd
Hertford Road
Hoddesdon
Hertfordshire
EN11 9BU
0992 467272

Merrell Dow Pharmaceuticals Ltd
Lakeside House
Stockley Park
Uxbridge
Middlesex
UB11 1BE
081 848 3456

Norwich Eaton Ltd
P O Box 1 YD
City Road
Newcastle upon Tyne
NE99 1YD
091 222 1882

Pharmax Ltd
Bourne Road
Bexley
Kent
DA5 1NX
0322 91321

Roche Products Ltd
P O Box 8
Welwyn Garden City
Hertfordshire
AL7 3AY
0707 328128

Roussel Laboratories Ltd
Broadwater Park
North Orbital Road
Denham
Uxbridge
Middlesex
UB9 5HP
0895 834343

Sandoz Pharmaceuticals
Frimley Business Park
Frimley
Camberley
Surrey
GU16 5SG
0276 692255

Sanofi UK Ltd
Floats Road
Wythenshawe
Manchester
M23 9NF
061 945 4161

Schwarz Pharma
Schwarz House
East Street
Chesham
Bucks
HP5 1DG
0494 772071

SmithKline Beecham Pharmaceuticals
Mundells
Welwyn Garden City
Hertfordshire
AL7 1EY
0707 325111

Stuart Pharmaceuticals
Stuart House
50 Alderley Road
Wilmslow
Cheshire
SK9 1RE
0625 535999

Tillotts Laboratories Ltd
see Farmitalia Carlo Erba Ltd

Wellcome Medical Division
Crewe Hall
Crewe
Cheshire
CW1 1UB
0270 583151

Wyeth Laboratories
Huntercombe Lane South
Maidenhead
Berks
SL6 0PH
0628 604377